Drug Discovery and Development

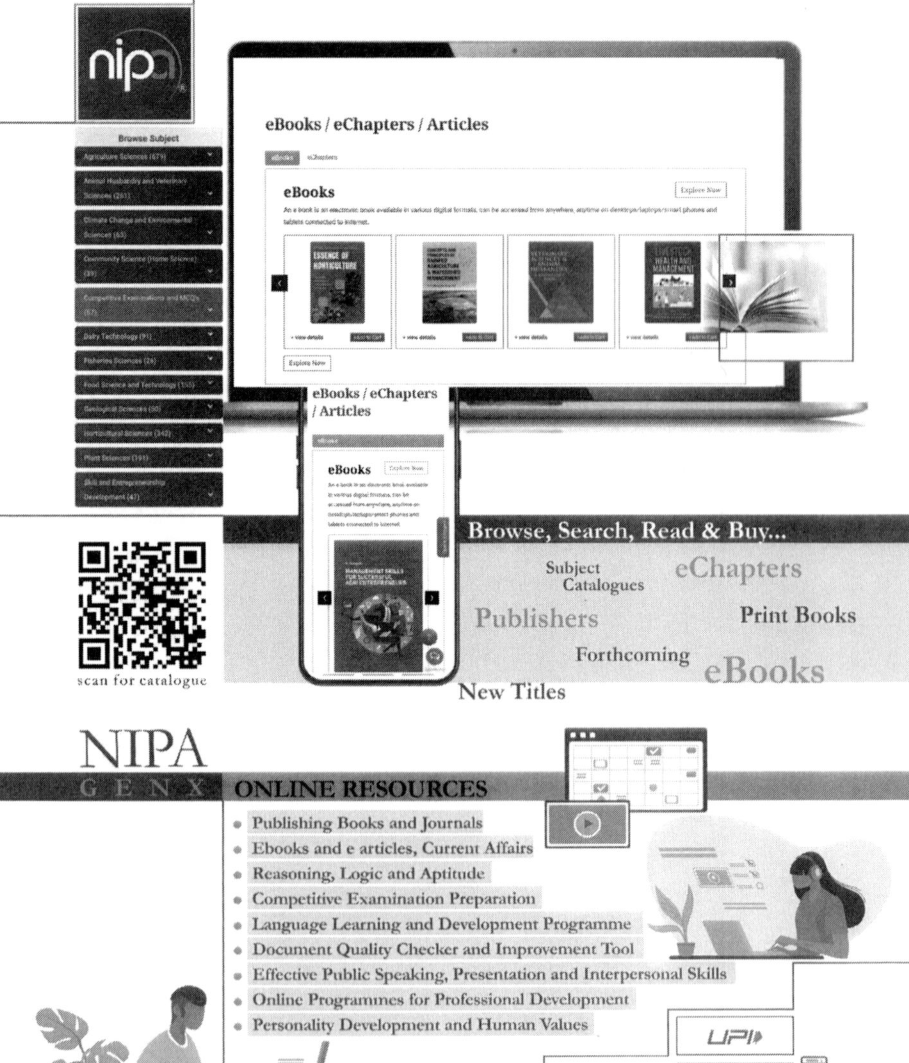

nipa
Browse Subject
eBooks / eChapters / Articles
eBooks
Explore Now
eBooks / eChapters / Articles
eBooks
Browse, Search, Read & Buy...
Subject Catalogues
eChapters
Publishers
Print Books
Forthcoming
eBooks
New Titles
scan for catalogue
NIPA
GENX
ONLINE RESOURCES
Publishing Books and Journals
Ebooks and e articles, Current Affairs
Reasoning, Logic and Aptitude
Competitive Examination Preparation
Language Learning and Development Programme
Document Quality Checker and Improvement Tool
Effective Public Speaking, Presentation and Interpersonal Skills
Online Programmes for Professional Development
Personality Development and Human Values
UPI
PayPal
PAY USING

Drug Discovery & Development

Traditional Medicine and Ethnopharmacology

BHUSHAN PATWARDHAN
Professor and Director
Interdisciplinary School of Health Sciences
University of Pune
Pune - 411 007, Maharashtra
INDIA

New India Publishing Agency
Pitam Pura, New Delhi- 110 088

Published by
Sumit Pal Jain *for*
New India Publishing Agency
101, Vikas Surya Plaza, CU Block, L.S.C. Mkt.,
Pitam Pura, New Delhi- 110 088, (India)
Phone: 011-27341717, Fax: 011-27341616
E-mail: newindiapublishingagency@gmail.com
Web: www.bookfactoryindia.com

ISBN : 81-89422-29-4

Composed and Designed by NIPA

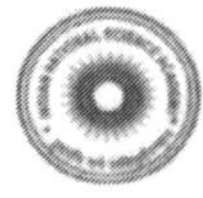

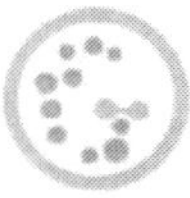

R A Mashelkar, FRS
Bhatnagar Fellow

President
Indian National Science Academy

President
Global Research Alliance

National Chemical Laboratory
Dr. Homi Bhabha Road, Pashan, Pune - 411 008. India

FOREWORD

There is a renewed interest now in ethnopharmacology and traditional medicine due to several reasons, including the serious innovation deficit faced by the industry and the escalating costs of putting molecules into the market place. Furthermore, in the present scenario, it has become important to understand the process of drug discovery development with a focus on herbal drugs and nutraceuticals.

It is being increasingly recognized that ethopharmacology, which largely uses natural materials such as herbs and minerals, can contribute as a discovery engine to provide new leads and also offer quality assured and standardized traditional medicines.

There is a clear movement to build a golden triangle between traditional medicine, modern medicine and modern science. This has had several fall outs. For example, the standard development route so far was "molecule to mice to men". We now have an alternative route of "men to mice to men", or in other words, "a reverse pharmacology route".

Interestingly enough, the discipline of pharmacognosy, as a science of crude drugs, has been transformed in to a new technology intensive multidisciplinary science.

The present book by Dr. Bhushan Patwardhan is absolutely timely, since it deals elegantly with all the above paradigm shifts in a cogent and comprehensive way.

The book is aptly divided in three parts. The first part covers the broad area of discovery including some key aspects of ethnopharmacology, bioprospecting, intellectual property rights, etc.

The second part covers the area of development including the pertinent safety and regulatory issues; quality control and standardization; stability and pharmacokinetics; preclinical and clinical evaluation; validation of health claims and pharmacoepidemiology, etc. There is some valuable guidance provided to the industry on regulatory issues.

The third part deals with the advent of new technology, and how it is influencing the whole process of discovery and development. The topics, among others, cover microarrays and high throughput screening; pharmacogenomics and ethopharmacology; ethoinformatics, etc. Excellent discussion on the system approach is also provided.

This book is valuable for the students and practitioners for a variety of reasons. Aspects of drug discovery, development and delivery have become important components of the pharmacy undergraduate and postgraduate programs all over the world.

The book gives excellent insights into good laboratory and good clinical practices. The processes involved in the filing of IND or NDA of botanical products along with a regulator's perspective of validating claims have been clearly explained. On a sound basis, it has been shown as to how an ethnopharmacological or traditional medicine needs to follow different approaches.

I am sure this book will serve as a most valuable resource for graduate and doctoral students in the field of pharmaceutical and health sciences. This is especially so for all those involved in drug research, clinical research or regulatory affairs related to ethnopharmacological, herbal, botanical, nutraceutical or such other natural medicines.

I wish to congratulate Dr. Bhushan Patwardhan for this wonderful book, which is based on his own experience in an area, in which he has himself made original contributions. I also congratulate New India Publishing Agency for publishing this book. I am sure this will be a valuable addition to the bookshelf of many practitioners and students, certainly it will be for mine.

R.A. Mashelkar

The University of Oxford

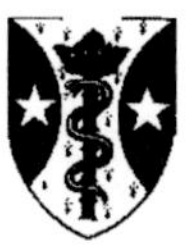

Green College
at the Radcliffe Observatory
Woodstock Road
Oxford. OX2 6HG

Telephone (01865) 274770
Fax. (01865) 274796

FELICITATIONS

June 2007

In the face of global demand for natural healthcare there is increased demand for products of a high standard of quality and safety.

Pharmacognosy, long a fading violet in the life sciences, has surged back into the frontline of research and development as this global trend for natural medicines expands. In the process, it has undergone enormous transformation from its early role as the science of drug development when most medicines were plant based. New technologies have evolved now to standardize plant-based medicines, ensure safety of both the product and the manufacturing process, and to determine efficacy. All of this is taking place against a regulatory backdrop which places high value on consumer safety.

The World Health Global Atlas on Traditional, Complementary & Alternative Medicine (Bodeker et al 2005) which my colleagues at Oxford and the London School of Hygiene and Tropical Medicine prepared for WHO in partnership with regional teams from around the world, indicated that the majority of the world's population is now using some form of natural healthcare on a regular basis. Within this trend, herbal medicine leads as an ever-expanding, global form of healthcare. Accordingly, it is natural for governments and international regulatory bodies to insist on high standards at every stage of the herbal drug manufacturing process. And it is equally reasonable for industry to expect that new graduates will be familiar with the latest technologies and methodologies for delivering these standards in their products.

Yet, the revitalized science of pharmacognosy - in support of its sister discipline of ethnopharmacology and in partnership with laboratory based natural products drug discovery - has been needing a standard reference. A single reference is needed to bring together all of the essential considerations, requirements, methodologies, awareness of regulatory policies and mastery of the latest technologies in order to equip industry, researchers and students with clear directions for proceeding at a high standard of quality and rigour.

Professor Bhushan Patwardhan's work has become well known internationally as presenting a high standard of evidence-based research on India's herbal heritage. He has also pioneered, with a group of distinguished colleagues, the new field of Ayurvedic Genomics – AyuGenomics, as it is now known – identifying a genetic basis to some central postulates in the classic texts of Ayurveda, India's time honoured system of natural healthcare.

This marriage of a high level of modern science with the deep insights into human functioning and of plant medicines, as described in ancient Ayurvedic science, has emerged as a vital and promising trend of 21st century India. A new generation of researchers now holds the promise of revealing, through the lens of modern science, the full potential of Ayurvedic knowledge, in company with the wisdom of India's other great traditions, including Unani and Siddha medicine, and other herbal traditions of the world.

Professor Bhushan's already important pioneering role in this revolution has been consolidated through the production of this very practical guide - a guide to the understanding and production of evidence-based herbal products as well as for leads for drug development. It is with high regard that I offer felicitations for this important work. This book will contribute seminally to the production of the new generation of researchers who will lead the revolution in healthcare, marrying the profound and life-supporting dimensions of ancient wisdom with the highest standards of modern science. Society at large will benefit.

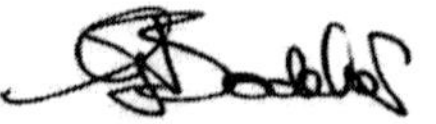

Dr. Gerard Bodeker
Division of Medical Sciences, University of Oxford, UK
& Adjunct Professor of Epidemiology, Mailman School of Public Health
Columbia University, New York, USA

Acknowledgement

This book is an outcome of group work of over 15 years and I thank each one of my students, associates and mentors who helped and guided me during this exciting journey of natural product: drug discovery and development. Many of my research associates and students have contributed by providing help in literature search and making useful notes. I specially mention Kalpana Joshi, Preeti Chavan (biotechnology, microarray), Yogita Ghodake (pharmacogenomics), Dyaneshwar Warude (quality, safety, and standardization), Girish Tillu (AyuSoft), Manish Gautam (pharmaceutics), Ashok Vaidya, Rama Vaidya and Amrutesh Puranik (history, reverse pharmacology, pharmacoepidemiology), Sanjay Mishra and Dada Patil (stability, preclinical). I wish to thank all the scientists and authors whose work has been cited in this book and also to various national and international bodies whose documents have been referred and cited including. I would like to especially mention the valuable resources from WHO, US FDA, ICH, ICMR, and CSIR. Much of the book is based on reviews published by our group in various Journals especially *Current Science, Journal of Ethnopharmacology, Evidence-based Complementary and Alternative Medicine, Journal of Scientific and Industrial Research, Indian Journal of Natural Products* and few of the studies I did for the WHO Commission on Intellectual Property Innovation and Public Health (CIPIH) and International Union of Pure and Applied Chemists (IUPAC). I wish to thank many who inspired and remained strong supporters specially Dr. R.A.

Mashelkar, Dr. Ashok Vaidya, Dr. G.N. Qazi, Dr. P. Pushpangadan, Dr. Arvind Chopra, Dr. Narendra Bhatt, Dr. Darshan Shankar, Dr. Mukund Chorghade, Dr. Avinash Patwardhan and Dr Alex Hankey.

A special appreciation and thanks to Ms Sarah Kimball, Rotary International Ambassadorial Scholar 2006-07 and a casual student of MPH course at the School of Health Sciences for valuable help in writing two chapters (Chapter 1 and 17) and also for thorough editing of the entire document.

I thank the authorities of the University of Pune for granting me a sabbatical leave that facilitated this book. A special thanks to the Manipal Group of Institutions for offering gracious Fellowship and hosting me at Manipal and Bangalore whenever required during the writing of this book. Finally, I wish to thank the entire management of New India Publishing Agency, New Delhi for suggesting, pursuing and also for accepting to publish this monumental work.

Bhushan Patwardhan

Pune

Contents

Part I : Discovery

1 Overview of Medical and Drug Development

To fully explore the history of medical and drug development, it would be necessary to go back as early as 13,000 BCE, where drawings on the Lascaux caves in France suggest that humans were using plants for medicinal purposes. Since then, medical traditions have evolved and dissolved across societies all over the globe. Natural products including plants, animals and minerals have been the basis of treatment of human diseases. The last two centuries have seen a focus on scientific medicine, with a focus on drugs whose effects that have been proved by the scientific method. Yet given this setting, many of the major pharmaceutical corporations have renewed their strategies in favor of natural product drug discovery. Numerous drugs have entered the international pharmacopoeia via the study of ethnopharmacology and traditional medicine. At this point in history, it is possible for both traditional and western medicine to benefit from collaboration between the two disciplines. For traditional medicines, newer guidelines of standardization, manufacture and quality control and scientifically rigorous research on the scientific basis for traditional treatments will be required. In return, traditional medical traditions can offer a more holistic approach to drug design and myriad possible targets for scientific analysis. Powerful new technologies such as automated separation techniques, high-throughput screening and combinatorial chemistry are revolutionizing drug discovery. Traditional knowledge can serve as powerful search engine, which will greatly facilitate intentional, focused and safe natural product drug discovery and help to rediscover the drug discovery process. By looking at the historical trends in drug and medical developments, it is possible to understand how current drug development will benefit from this partnership.

Historical Perspective of the Pharmaceutical Industry

Until World War II, German and Swiss chemical companies dominated the pharmaceutical industry. The war served as a powerful impetus for medical development, and many techniques followed that greatly improved the health conditions of the time, such as the ability to mass-produce penicillin, which made antibiotics readily available. Driven by the emergence of socialized medicine and a period of economic growth, German and Swiss companies synthesized a large number of anti-bacterial drugs and other compounds creating a prosperous market. The success of these firms was the result of growing expenditure for drugs in a free market, loose regulation regarding drug safety, patent protection in their country of origin, capital access and chemical process know-how from chemical business. Moreover, the absence of almost any drug before WWII facilitated the success of random screening drug discovery tools.

By the end of the 60's and beginning of 70's the industry begin to experience the crisis because of increasing R&D costs coupled with decreasing revenues. There were two main factors driving this increase in costs. One was the introduction of stricter regulations on drug safety, which resulted in both an increase in the cost and in the lengthening of clinical trials leading to longer time-to-market.

The second factor was the decreased profitability and substantial increase in R&D expenses as all obvious routes to new drugs on the basis of the chemical synthetic paradigm had been exploited. To aggravate the situation, many pharmaceutical companies emerged and started eroding the dominance of the Swiss-German firms' duopoly and many European countries introduced price control measures.

At about the same time, two new technological paradigms were beginning to emerge outside of the industry: biotechnology and bioinformatics. Bioinformatics focused on *improving random techniques* for testing new compounds by using High-Throughput Screening (HTS) tools, such as biochips, and combinatorial chemistry. Since then, these two techniques have allowed 7- folds increase in the number of compounds tested per year. Biotechnology focused on *rational drug design* by applying engineering and scientific principles to the processing of materials by biological agents. While biotechnology and bioinformatics may seem different in spirit, they were used synergistically. Biotechnology helped searching promising families of compounds among hundred of thousands of molecular entities and bioinformatics speeded up the testing of compounds of those families against a diverse number of diseases.

Despite the fact that both American and European pharmaceuticals were desperately trying to increase drug throughput into the market and these new paradigms promised a revolutionary shift, none of those firms took part in the initial development and commercialization of biotechnology. The economic reason was the large amount of capital investments necessary to develop biotechnology and bioinformatics in a period of cost containment for large pharmaceuticals. The structural reason was the revolutionary change in expertise involved with embracing biotechnology. One major aspect of biotechnology is its multidisciplinary character that draws on a new number of scientific disciplines including biology, biochemistry, genetics, microbiology, biochemical engineering and separation processing. For a large vertically integrated pharmaceutical firm, whose competence and success relied on developing and processing chemicals, this was simply an unthinkable organizational revolution.

The development of biotechnology in US rather than in Europe was the consequence of a set of regional advantages combined with governmental policies. Huge commitment came from the US government of federal funds to health and biotechnology research just at the time when the major breakthroughs in genetic engineering were being made. The US National Institute of Health (NIH), for example, invested in basic research at a much higher level than European governments. Figures indicate that in '70s and '80s the expenditure for health-related research of UK, France and Canada combined together was around 12-15% of the US level over the same period.

The *Bayh-Dole Act* in 1980 weakened ownership rights of public institutions, such as universities and national labs, over the research developed under their auspices. This facilitated the private appropriation and commercialization of publicly funded research and encouraged the transfer of patented technologies into entrepreneurial entities.

A set of new legislative decisions, such as the biotech patent (1983), which reinforced and expanded property rights for biotech products, and the Orphan Drug Act (1984), which subsidized the research for rare diseases, created the premises for the creation of Dedicated Biotechnology Firms (DBFs). The fact that these companies could rely on royalties from patents as a secure source of income was a strong driving force that gave the impetus for companies to engage in research.

The strong US venture capital market, stimulated by this new legislative environment, provided the necessary capital for these new DBFs. At the same time, venture capitalists provided managerial and business expertise, which many of these pure research-oriented companies were lacking, by nominating some of their representatives onto the companies boards. The well-developed secondary stock markets in the US offered an additional resource of capital for growing company. Stock options served as a very strong incentive for attracting human capital from universities or national labs. All these factors worked synergistically in the US, and by the mid 80's, biotechnology was an established sector in the pharmaceutical industry.

By the early '80's large pharmaceutical firms, which deliberately did not invest in biotech in the '70's, recognized that this new technology was sufficiently mature and would be essential for future product innovation. However, these companies pursued different strategies and moved at different speed to embrace biotechnology. Some companies decided to build new competencies through the acquisition of DBFs, others through merger with US counterparts, and some others through external linkages with US and/or European DBFs. For example, Welcome, Galax and Bayer chose to link up directly with their corporate US laboratories; ICI (later Zeneca) opted for reinforcing its link with the UK science; Hoechst, Ciba Geigy and Hoffmann LaRoche placed more emphasis on research alliances with DBFs. Bayer, Montedison and other German and Italian firms embraced biotechnology later, probably because their natural tendency to rely on chemicals as their core competencies. At the same time, large firms increased the practice of contracting out some of the more routine aspects of R&D activities in the pre-clinical and clinical trials to contract research organizations (CROs). While the emergence of DBFs and CROs did not weakened in any significant way the power of the large established firms, they started changing the internal organization of large pharmaceuticals and shifting the competitive advantage from large vertically integrated firms to large flexible and interconnected firms.

In the '90s, the US pharmaceutical market has grown from being roughly equal to the European market to almost twice as much, representing today 40% the total world sales. Even more shocking is that the US market alone accounts for 60% of total worldwide company profits. This dramatic change forced European companies to increase competitiveness on the North American market in order to benefit from larger profits. This competitiveness was pursued via a process of decentralization, mergers, acquisitions, and specialization. First, many large European chemical conglomerates, such as the German Hoechst and the Swiss ICI, de-merged their pharmaceutical subsidiaries from their bulk chemical activities, realizing that at this point was more a burden than an advantage. Secondly, many large firms merged to increase penetration in US and to leverage economy of scale on R&D: Glaxo and Wellcome merged in 1995; Sandoz and Ciba-Geigy formed Novartis in 1996; Astra and Zeneca merged in 1998; Hoechst and Rhone-Poulenc formed Aventis in 1999. Finally, many of these firms started specializing on a particular area of pharmaceutical research, such as cardiovascular or neural-system drugs, and developed strong collaboration in world regions that excel in that area.

The results of this historical confluence explain several important elements of the current scenario of pharmaceutical companies. The emergence of biotechnology firms in US was not the result of direct intervention of large pharmaceutical firms, but the synergistic consequence of governmental policies and the entrepreneurial nature of US market. Biotechnology has not displaced the power of large pharmaceutical firms, as many like to think, but it has changed their internal organization in a revolutionary way. The industry is shifting from large vertically integrated pharmaceutical firms to horizontally specialized DBFs and CROs coordinated by large flexible pharmaceutical firms.

The strategies of the European pharmaceutical firms of moving R&D to US and M&A are dictated by the necessity to compete with global markets.

Ethnopharmacology and Natural Products (NP)

The investigation of natural products as source of novel human therapeutics reached its peak in the Western pharmaceutical industry during 1970–1980, which resulted in a pharmaceutical landscape heavily influenced by non-synthetic molecules. Of the 877 small-molecule NCE introduced between 1981 and 2002, roughly half (49%) were NP, semi-synthetic NP analogues or synthetic compounds based on NP. In terms of the number of species individually targeted, the use of plants as medicines represents by far the biggest human use of the natural world. There is no reliable figure for the total number of medicinal plants on Earth, and numbers and percentages for countries and regions vary greatly. Estimates for the numbers of species used medicinally include: 35,000-70,000 or 53,000 worldwide; 10,000-11,250 in China, 7500 in India and 2572 traditionally by North American Indians. The number of plant species that provide ingredients for drugs used in Western Medicine is even fewer. It was calculated for an article published in 1991 that there were 121 drugs in current use in the USA derived from plants, with 95 species acting as sources (more than one drug is obtained from some species). Despite the small number of source species, drugs derived from plants are of immense importance in terms of numbers of patients treated. It is reported that 25% of all prescriptions dispensed from community pharmacies in the USA between 1959 and 1973 contained one or more ingredients derived from higher plants. A more recent study, of the top 150 proprietary drugs used in the USA in 1993, found that 57% of all prescriptions contained at least one major active compound currently or once derived from (or patterned after) compounds derived from biological diversity.

Financially, the retail sales of pharmaceutical products were estimated at US$ 80-90 billion globally in 1997, with medicinal plants contributing very significantly. A study of the 25 best-selling pharmaceutical drugs in 1997 found that 11 of them (42%) were biologicals, natural products or entities derived from natural products, with a total value of US$ 17.5 billion. The total sales' value of drugs (such as Taxol) derived from just one plant species (*Taxus baccata*) was US$ 2.3 billion in 2000. The world market for herbal remedies in 1999 was estimated to be worth US$ 19.4 billion, with Europe leading (US$ 6.7 billion), followed by Asia (US$ 5.1 billion), North America (US$ 4.0 billion), Japan (US$ 2.2 billion), and then the rest of the world (US$ 1.4 billion).

There is a good deal of trade in NP, on scales ranging from the local to the international. Much of this is unrecorded in official statistics or poorly documented, which explains why there is typically so little awareness among decision-makers of the significance of the trade to the healthcare and economies of their people, or about problems of unsustainability and the sometimes-deleterious impacts of wild collection on natural habitats. Large quantities of NP are traded into urban centers from rural areas in developing countries, and also regionally and internationally. China's production of medicinal plants from cultivated and wild-harvested sources, considered together, was calculated at 1.6 million tonnes in 1996, with a total value (excluding exports) in terms of finished products of US$ 3.7 billion. The reported annual imports of NP material into all countries during the 1990s amounted to an average of 400,000 tonnes, valued at US$ 1.2 billion, showing a 100% rise between 1991 and 1997. The three leading exporting countries are China (ca. 140,000 tonnes per year over 1991-1997), India (about one-third of the Chinese amount) and then Germany. Europe is the major trading centre for MAPs globally, with imports into one European country or another amounting to 440,000 tonnes in 1996. There are at least 2000 species of NP marketed in Europe originating from over 120 countries. It is guessed that the total number of NP in international trade may be about 2500 species.

Although the vastness of these numbers suggests that there is a wide scope of people who benefit from medicinal plants, it is typically the poorest who are the most dependent on medicinal plants because they are often the only affordable and culturally acceptable option. Only 15% of pharmaceutical drugs are consumed in developing countries, and a large proportion of even this small percentage is taken by the more affluent sector. The dried plants that are used as herbal medicines in urban centers are collected from rural areas. In this way, medicinal plants can provide a significant source of income for rural people in developing countries, especially through the sale of wild-harvested material. The collectors are often herders, shepherds or other economically marginalized sections of the population, such as landless people and women. Between 50-100% of households in the northern part of central Nepal and about 25-50% in the middle part of the same region are involved in collecting medicinal plants for sale in the wholesale markets in Delhi. The money received represents 15-30% of the total income of poorer households. Medicinal plants can also be symbolically very important to people. They can be held in special religious, nationalistic or ideological esteem. This can also carries challenges, in that this allegiance to medicinal plants can prevent people from accepting equally or more effective substitutes, and uncompromising attitudes towards the ownership of the plants and who should benefit from (or pay for) their continuing existence. Although, botanical medications continued to be produced in every country, the variance between varieties usually is not evaluated and the composition of these complex mixtures has only crudely analyzed.

Ayurvedic Indian and traditional Chinese systems are living great traditions. These traditions have relatively organized database, and more exhaustive description of botanical material that is available and can be tested using modern scientific methods. Both systems of medicine thus have an important role in bioprospecting of new medicines. Good botanical practices which can improve the quality control procedures of monitoring impurities, heavy metals and other toxins in the raw material can make the NP research more meaning full.

Modern techniques like HTS and combinatorial chemistry are making the DD programmes more technology driven. The computer-based design of hit and lead structure candidates emerged as a complementary approach to high-throughput screening. The goal of current DD aims to create a single chemical substance which will interact specifically with a single molecular target to perturb *in vivo* biochemistry in a way that eliminates the biochemical changes that are the consequence of the disease, reinstating healthy-state biochemistry. The serendipitous approach consequently turned in to target-centric DD, practiced intensely by pharmaceutical companies for the past 30 years. This approach was successful for the past thirty years, which saw the understanding and development of methods to isolate and study molecules, cells and other components of living system. With the completion of the HGP at the end of 20th century, public sector researchers - spurred in part by various NIH Initiatives - focused in DD and development of new chemical entities. HGP inspired the idea of so called a 'druggable genome'[3] and bioinformatics approaches offered large and diverse chemical libraries that could be readily screened on targets offered by HGP. But transforming these chemical libraries into drugs remains a challenging endeavor. Despite the predicted increase in potential new drug targets for different diseases, there is currently a dearth of new drugs. Molecules designed to interact with a single target often have unanticipated effects on 'off target' biochemical mechanisms and the safety implications of those unwanted effects might not be revealed until a drug candidate is in large-scale clinical trials or even on the market.

Drug Discovery (DD) in current scenario has become unproductive to the point where the economic future of the industry is questionable. To push into the future, the R&D thrust in the pharmaceutical sector needs to be focused on development of new drugs, innovative processes for known drugs and development of plant-based drugs through investigation of leads from the traditional systems of medicine. Traditional medicine can provide novel inputs into the drug development process. For instance, a consortium led by the Medical Research Council of South Africa is carrying out a study on traditional medicines used by communities for the self-treatment of fevers, with the aim of discovering active compounds to treat malaria more effectively. Other cases have highlighted the possibility that traditional medicines and natural products may be used as a source of drugs designed principally to meet the needs of developed country markets (e.g. appetite suppressants). At the same time "bioprospecting"— the search for economically valuable natural resources – by pharmaceutical companies, or on their behalf, has not been conspicuously successful in recent years. Various institutions, including the Council for Scientific and Industrial Research (CSIR) in India, are taking another tack, exploring alternative paths to modern pharmaceutical research presented by traditional medicine—paths that could be cheaper, faster and more effective. One such strategy involves a process known as "reverse pharmacology", which begins with a useful natural product and works backward, as it were, to identify its active ingredients. CSIR has begun clinical trials on herbal products of medicinal value generated through reverse pharmacology, with several public and private partners. In looking to the future, it is important to consider the relative potential of these approaches to generating cost-effective, safe medical products.

❑❑❑

2 TM / CAM and Ethnopharmacology

Historically, the terms alternative, complementary or traditional medicine (TM) all referred to a genre of health care practices or services that got bound together as a class through the logic of reductio-ad-absurdum, or because of their "absence from the mainframe of" what has come to be known as Modern Medicine (MM). However, since Stephen Fulder[1], the identities of TM have become more distinct, MM-TM blending more active and, the line separating the two more fuzzy. To date, the World Health Organization offers the most comprehensive definition of TM[2].

WHO defines traditional medicine as including diverse health practices, approaches, knowledge and beliefs incorporating plant, animal, and/or mineral based medicines, spiritual therapies, manual techniques and exercises applied singularly or in combination to maintain well-being, as well as to treat, diagnose or prevent illness.

The phraseology MM/TM is syntactically incorrect because it is contended that medicine as such, modern or otherwise, evolves and progresses through traditions. The major difference between the various traditions of health

[1] Fulder S. Handbook of Complementary and Alternative Medicine.

[2] WHO Traditional Medicine Strategy 2002-2005, WHO Geneva, 2002.

care practices is that MM rode the crest of the high wave of reductionist-scientistic rigor of modernity[3] to reach the shore of global acceptability while the others never crossed the threshold of geographical and cultural locality, remaining untested, neither proved nor disproved. Darwinian principle of survival of the fittest also endorses a truism that survival is a proof of fitness. Given this principle, it makes sense that TM as we know of it today may be useful for promoting human health. Moreover, most TM considers human beings and their health in the context of their environment. This criteria, not only defines TM apart from MM but also provides for a reason as to why lately TM is emerging out of long hibernation. Developmentally, MM isolated "human" from its global environmental context as a static, stand-alone, complete, total and delimited system in itself. While this reductionist approach has a very high pay off for the first 90% of human health problems, it fails when dynamic non-linear complex systems elements kick in (I'm not exactly sure that you mean by this phrase). TM covers some parts of those hidden variables and thats the utility to modern mankind.

Traditional Medicine (TM) and Complementary and Alternative Medicine (CAM) are attracting more and more global attention within the context of health care provision and health sector reform. Many factors are contributing to widespread interest in TM/CAM. But if their potential is to be developed successfully, some important issues must be addressed. TM is a comprehensive term used to refer both to TM systems such as traditional Chinese medicine, Indian Ayurveda, Arabic Unani medicine, and to various forms of indigenous medicine. TM therapies can include medication therapies if they involve the use of herbal medicines, animal parts and/or minerals, and non-medication therapies if they are carried out primarily

[3] Age of Enlightenment, Age of Reason (AD 1600- AD 1900).

without the use of material medicines, as in the case of acupuncture, manual therapies and spiritual therapies. In countries where the dominant health care system is based on allopathic medicine, or where TM has not been incorporated into the national health care system, TM is often termed "complementary", "alternative" or "non-conventional" medicine.

Throughout history, Asian, African, Arabic, Native American, Oceanic, Central and South American and other cultures have developed a variety of indigenous TM systems. Influenced by factors such as history, personal attitudes and philosophy, their practices vary greatly across different countries and regions.Their theory and application often differ significantly from those of allopathic medicine. Traditional medicine may be codified, regulated, taught openly and practiced widely and systematically, and many benefit from thousands of years of experience. Conversely, some traditions are highly secretive, mystical and extremely localized, with knowledge of its practices passed on orally. It may be based on salient physical symptoms or perceived supernatural forces. Clearly, at global level, traditional medicine eludes precise definition or description, as it containsdiverse and sometimes conflicting characteristics and viewpoints.

Distinct ustoms of TM are as numerous as the geographical and cultural contexts were that gave birth to them. Interplay between geography and evolution is well known[4] . Geography, not only shapes human social cultures, but it also influences vastly the biosphere and its ecology in any given region. Whether the distinctiveness and diversity of TM is a merit or a demerit depends on the perspective of medical science. While 99+% of the human biology is the same all across the planet there is some minor but

---

[4] "Guns, Germs, and Steel: The Fates of Human Societies": Jared Diamond.

nonetheless distinct and unique element of variability in human biology.

Acupuncture is a traditional Chinese medicinal therapy. But many European countries define it and traditional Chinese medicine in general as CAM, because it is not included in their own health care traditions. Similarly, since homeopathy and chiropractic systems were developed in Europe in the 18th Century, after the introduction of allopathic medicine, they are not categorized as TM systems nor incorporated into the dominant modes of health care in Europe. Instead, they are regarded as a form of CAM. Accordingly, in this document, "traditional medicine" is used when referring to Africa, Latin America, South-East Asia, and/or the Western Pacific, whereas "complementary and alternative medicine" is used when referring to Europe and/or North America (and Australia). When referring in a general sense to all of these regions, the comprehensive TM/CAM is used.

Diversity and Distinctiveness

World Health Organization has defined three types of health systems to describe the degree to which TM/CAM is an officially recognized element of healthcare. In an integrative system, TM/CAM is officially recognized and incorporated into all areas of health care provision. This means that TM/CAM is included in the relevant country's national drug policy; providers and products are registered and regulated; TM/CAM therapies are available at hospitals and clinics (both public and private); treatment with TM/CAM is reimbursed under health insurance; relevant research is undertaken; and education in TM/CAM is available. Worldwide, only China, the Democratic People's Republic of Korea, the Republic of Korea and Vietnam can be considered to have attained an integrative system.

An inclusive system recognizes TM/CAM, but has not yet fully integrated it into all aspects of health care, be this health care delivery, education and training, or regulation. Under these systems, TM/CAM is not be available at all health care levels, health insurance is not cover treatment with TM/CAM, official education in TM/CAM is not be available at university level, and regulation of TM/CAM providers and products is lacking or only partial. That said, work on policy, regulation, practice, health insurance coverage, research and education is under way. Countries operating an inclusive system include developing countries such as India, Equatorial Guinea, Nigeria and Mali which have a national TM/CAM policy, but little or no regulation of TM/CAM products, and developed countries such as Canada and the United Kingdom which do not offer significant University-level education in TM/CAM, but which are making concerted efforts to ensure the quality and safety of TM/CAM. Ultimately, countries operating an inclusive system can be expected to attain an integrative system. Lastly, in countries with a tolerant system, the national health care system is based entirely on allopathic medicine, although the law recognizes some TM/CAM practices as legitimate.

Healthcare Delivery and Treatments

There are different needs and driving forces that make consumers seek for TM based health care delivery and treatments. WHO believes that consumer information and education will help consumers to seek out appropriate types of self-care and as a result, help them to obtain more benefits from TM/ CAM and reduce unnecessary risks. Studies show that many patients use TM/CAM therapies concurrently with conventional medicine, often without informing their health care provider, which can potententially cause harm to the patient if the therapies contradict each other. It is essential for the safety of patients that consumer information is available about TM/CAM so that they can make educated choices about their own health care consumption. TM/CAM is unregulated in most countries, communication between patients and health care providers is generally poor, and there is an urgent need to develop consumer information in order to minimize the risks and maximize the benefits of TM/CAM use[5].

A WHO data query engine shows the density of physicians (Modern Medicine) per 100,000 persons in various countries (up to date as of 2004) as: Rwanda 1.87, Ethiopia 2.85, Uganda 4.70, Benin 5.75, India 51.25 and China 164.24 (in contrast the numbers for Australia and the USA are 249.13 and 548.91 respectively). These data show the under served the health care needs in developing countries. Against this background, we see that in Tanzania Uganda and Zambia the ratio of TM practitioners[6] is between 400 and 500 per 100,000 persons (still less than but comparable to the number of modern medicine physicians available to the USA population) and the number of TM practitioners in Sub Saharan Africa is 100 times that of the modern medicine physicians. It should come as no surprise that 70% Rwandans, 90% Ethiopians, 60% Ugandans, 80% Beninans, 70% Indians and, 40% Chinese among the developing countries[7] use TM as a means to their Health care needs[8].

---

[5] Zhang, Xiaorui Department of Essential Drugs and Medicines Policy, WHO Guidelines on Developing Consumer Information on Proper Use of Traditional,Complementary and Alternative Medicine, 2004, World Health Organization, Geneva.

[6] World Health Organization Traditional Medicine Strategy 2002-2005, WHO Geneva.

[7] The explanation to the paradox, why 48% Australians and 42% USA citizens have used TM at least once will be addressed later.

[8] WHO TM Strategy 2002-2005.

The last hundred years have brought forth major advances in science and technology at the service of human kind and yet we have failed to make these magnificent advances accessible, available and affordable with decent equity to all. The world stands more divided and more polarized than ever before and this chasm is widening at an alarming pace. While creativity and talent reinforcement by technological resources seem poised to soar towards unprecedented heights, suddenly we find ourselves confronted and constrained by the old ghouls of wars, pandemics, and poverty that for a brief while we thought we had left behind for good. Moreover, the paradox is that this discomforting reality has afflicted even the rich and the privileged. Leaders, policy makers, and scholars all over the world over are grappling with solutions to these complex problems - because there is no single magic bullet, no single solution. This report, within the paradigm of health, but against the backdrop of the philosophical underpinnings outlined above, tries to explore the place and utility of Traditional Medicine as a vehicle to affordable health to large un-served or underserved population in the developing countries.

While the global village is stuck at a bottleneck regarding equity of distribution of modern medicine, modern science is stuck at another stagnation - a bottleneck of innovation. Despite the availability of humungous data and resources, newer innovative discoveries are not pouring in at the expected high rates, tipping the benefit cost ratio to an alarming low. The situation seems to demand rejuvenation.. It may be possible to remedy this situation through collaboration of TM/CAM and MM, using TM/CAM as a starting place for drug discovery.

It is argued that TM runs afoul in the areas of validity and verfiability. Broadly the deficiencies in TM can be categorized as: Lack of validation, Lack of standardization, Lack of delivery infrastructure, Lack of integration- intra or interdisciplinary. If we analyze undercurrents that fuel these lacunae we see main two - poverty and policy. Poverty, directly connected to the issue of affordability of health care, is the prime cause of use, misuse and abuse of Traditional Medicine. If there were no poverty in the developing countries, modern medicine would have undoubtedly rendered TM extinct through Darwinian processes. Poverty also has provoked abuse of TM by charlatans that in turn feeds into skepticism and cynicism about TM in the mind of scholars and policy makers. It would be unfortunate to allow those who are exploiting people by mimicking TM to invalidate the entire field. Unless the vicious circle of poverty is broken, health care standards for the underprivileged in the world cannot be raised, nor can what that is good in TM can be salvaged and used to further modern medicine.

To bring affordable and efficacious health care to the population in the developing world, local governments' and international agencies' involvement is of paramount importance. Given that TM can serve as a cheap and culturally acceptable form of health care, prime issues of concern for attention of local government and/or policy makers are: endorsement of TM, validation of efficacy, regulation of safety, standardization of materials and harmonization of practices, professionals' training, construction of delivery infrastructure, protection of intellectual property, enforcement of equitable distribution of TM, guarantee of sustainability of supply of resources, supervision of price structure, Intellectual Property Rights (IPR) inequities and back pressure from pharmaceutical industries (lack of innovations and productive outcomes). This makes new approaches such as Reverse Pharmacology and Systems Biology more attractive because they provide innovation opportunities that are based on experiential wisdom and the holistic viewpoint of TM. Current policies on IPR at an international level are detrimental to making health care available and affordable to developing countries and therefore the *sue generis* systems become more important to protect interests of the traditional knowledge from possible exploitations. While new drug discovery slows down, reducing profits from western market, pharmaceuticals are not only in a defensive turf battle posture at home but are applying rules of the game uniformly to uneven playfields. This makes medicines unaffordable to the developing countries while at the same time hurts the corporations by making them lose the partial gain that they could make by flexing to accommodate economic limitations of the developing world. Given that they would need to compete with the same large pharmaceutical companies, it is understandably that TM would be put into a defensive secretive mode that diminishes innovative original ideas flowing from TM to modern medicine.

The advantages of TM include its widespread accessibility and relative affordability, which is particularly important because most people in low-income countries pay for medicines out of their own pockets. The governments of China and India, amongst others, provide governmental support to strengthen training, research and the use of "traditional" medicine in their national healthcare strategies, and a number of African countries are considering how to integrate traditional medicine into "mainstream" healthcare[9]. The possibilities for expanding such initiatives need to be examined. Apart from medical use, the production, sale and export of traditional medicines is an important component in some economies. China, for

[9] Kimani Chege, Kenya to develop traditional medicine action plan, 29 June 2004, SciDev.Net.

instance, exports over $600 million of traditional medicine products annually. Chinese health authorities have recently launched a nationwide program to build up 161 Traditional Chinese medicine (TCM) hospitals, each specializing in the treatment of a particular condition, such as different types of cancers, heart and vascular diseases and hepatitis[10].

Traditional medicines may have been used for centuries by communities who have found them to be efficacious through experience. But their mode of action may not be understood in modern scientific terms, and they often consist of mixtures of different active substances. This makes it very difficult for them to be subjected to analysis by the methods of modern science, or to meet the regulatory and approval mechanisms designed for single molecule modern medicines. This means that the efficacy of traditional approaches has generally not been described in terms of contemporary regulatory standards of the developed world. This has implications for certifying their quality, and for promoting their use outside the communities from which they originate. WHO reports that a growing number of countries are adopting national policies and developing specific regulatory capacity on traditional medicine; moreover, there is strong scientific evidence for some traditional approaches like acupuncture.

Nevertheless, there continue to be considerable challenges, including the varying degree to which traditional approaches are recognized by governments, lack of scientific evidence on efficacy, and difficulties in assuring proper use. A particular feature of traditional medicines is that they are based on natural products. Expanding their use therefore may depend on ensuring sustainable supplies of natural raw materials, and consideration of the economics

---

[10] Jia Hepeng, China to boost traditional medicine hospitals 2 July 2004, Sci Dev.Nett.

of production and processing, and the implications for the availability and cost of the finished product. Also, as natural products, there may be challenges in ensuring consistency and stability in the product. The study should consider the specific policy and regulatory issues regarding traditional medicine, and their interaction with the systems designed for modern medicine.

Health Needs of Developing Countries

Developing countries lately have come to be identified and distinguished from the developed world through three key characteristics: disproportionate population growth, disproportionate affliction with mainly infectious diseases and, health care that is increasingly out of reach for most of their inhabitants. The world has reached a population of approximately 6.4 billion[11] as this report is being written. Out of these about 81.8% lives in the developing countries[12]. An estimated 7.4 million people are living with HIV in China, Indonesia and Vietnam, 5.1 million in India alone, 1.6 million in Latin America and, 25 million people in sub-Saharan Africa[13]. In contrast an estimated mere 1.6 million people are living with HIV in developed countries all together. There are at least 300 million acute cases of malaria each year globally, resulting in more than a million deaths. Around 90% of these deaths occur in Africa, mostly in young children[14]. Against that, malaria is virtually non-existent in developed world. The number of persons who suffered from Tuberculosis (all forms) in 2002[15] was 532 per 100,000

---

[11] U.S. Bureau of the Census.

[12] Based on United Nations, World Population Prospects, The 1998 Revision; and estimates by the Population Reference Bureau.

[13] UNAIDS 2004 Report on the Global AIDS Epidemic - Executive Summary.

[14] Roll Back Malaria (a global partnership initiated by WHO, UNDP, UNICEF and the World Bank) fact sheet.

[15] WHO Fact Sheet N 104 revised March 2004.

in Africa and South East Asia put together, out of which 122 died. However, in America and Europe the respective numbers were 97 and 14. In 2000, while average per capita spending on pharmaceuticals in high-income countries was $400, it was barely over $4 in low-income countries. At the extremes of the spectrum of the data the difference was 1,000 fold. Moreover, in 2003, while the estimated cost of treatment for HIV/AIDS was $300 plus per annum, in eight of the 23 countries that make up 80% of the global treatment need, the average spending on the pharmaceutical was $5 per head in 2000[16]. This data shows how badly under served the health care needs in developing countries are.

While it could be argued that these problems in developing countriesare of their own making and need local fixes, they truly are a matter of global concern. The health problems of the developing world, if left unreconciled or unresolved could push humanity beyond the tipping point, with dire unprecedented consequences for all humanity, sparing and forgiving none- neither developing nor developed countries. Global wars and terrorism make two glaring examples of the outcomes that can happen when countries alienate each other and fail to collaborate.

Statistics that evaluate health measures paint a dire picture. Over one billion people exist on less than one dollar a day. The world population has increased from approximately 2.8 billion to currently in excess of 6.3 billion and today over 2.5 billion people lack sanitation, over 1.5 billion people do not have safe drinking water, and some 3 million people, mostly women and children, die every year from diarrheal diseases directly related to these deficiencies. There is little cause for optimism in these areas: indeed, available evidence suggests that the availability of water in

[16] World Medicine Situation, 2004, a WHO report.

the poor world is likely to diminish rather than increase over the next several decades[17]. The importance of a public health infrastructure cannot be overemphasized: the increase in life expectancy during the 20th century was due in significant part to public health services, including sanitation, cleaner water, mass vaccinations, and improved workplace safety[18,19,20].

It is true that what you really value is what you miss, not what you have[21]. TM has become an extremely valuable commodity for the world today, precisely because it provides what the world misses most. The low-income developing countries miss the modern medicine because they cannot afford it whereas high-income developed world misses the holistic wisdom implicit in TM.

Ayurveda – The Ancient Science of Life

Currently, with over 400,000 registered Ayurveda practitioners, Government of India has formal structures to regulate issues related to quality, safety, efficacy and practice of herbal medicine[22]. With a unique holistic approach, Ayurvedic medicines are usually customized to an individual based on their constitution. Ayurvedic philosophy strongly believes that human being is a microcosm of nature and all the five basic elements of nature are present in him.

---

[17] Aldhous P. 2003. The world's forgotten crisis. Nature 422:251–253.

[18] Triggle D. Medicines in the 21st Century. DRUG DEVELOPMENT RESEARCH 59:269–291 (2003)

[19] Longman PJ. 2003. The health of nations. Wash Monthly April:16–23.

[20] Hertzman C. 2001. Health and human society. Am Scientist Nov/ Dec:538–545.

[21] Jorge Luis Borges

[22] National Policy on Indian Systems of Medicine and Homoeopathy-2002, Ministry of Health and Family Welfare, Government of India <www.indianmedicine.nic.in>.

The original philosophical basis of Ayurveda is in Sankhya, which means "knowing the truth". Sankhya is the philosophy of creation and is based on the twenty four principles or elements of the universe. Prakruti is a female principle and Purusha is a male principle and together they evolve Mahad - universal intellect. Its first manifestation is Ahamkar or Ego, which further manifests into five basic principles or Panchamahabhootas. This is the basic concept of Ayurvedic philosophy. Some of the fundamentals of Ayurvedic philosophy are outlined below:

Five basic elements of nature are called as Panch (five) Maha (great) Bhootas (elements). These Panchamahaboota include: Earth (Pruthvi), Water (Aap), Fire (Tejas), Air (Vayu) and Ether (Akash). Earth element relates to sense of smell, Water relates to taste, Fire relates to vision, Air relates to touch and Ether relates to hearing. Thus these five elements are connected with five sensory organs: ear, tongue, eye, skin and nose respectively. These five elements in various permutations and combination proportions form all living bodies including the human. Therefore every human being has its own character presented in form of its Prakruti or Constitution - some thing like a genetic structure determined at the time of birth.

The five Panchamahabhoota in the human body and their combination proportions determine the constitution or Prakruti of that individual and is presented in form of Tri-Doshas or three humors, Vata (Air and Ether), Pitta (Fire and Water) and Kapha (Water and Earth). Water predominates in the overall constitution of human body as it is part of Kapha and Pitta constitution. There are three main constitutions, seven types of secondary and many subtle combinations of Vata, Pitta, Kapha (VPK) depending on the individual proportions. As per the Ayurvedic principles, an individual is born with a definite Prakruti, which remains unaltered throughout the life span quite similar to the genome. However, the combination of the basic elements that govern patho-physiological changes in the body can alter its response due to variety of causative factors including diet, environment, life-style, infection and like. Disease prevention and health promotion through the use of Ayurvedic therapeutics revolves around obtaining back the original balance of the basic elements by manipulations of materials and procedures so as to remove imbalance of Tri-Dosha.

Human constitution or Prakruti can be determined and wide spectrums of indicators are available for this purpose. These indicators are based on a patient's past history; observations, physical examination, psychological profile, and social, cultural, ethnic aspects also serve as compounding factors. Since this determination of Prakruti has subjective considerations of individual and physician, it might vary due to differences in their understanding. However, attempts have been made to bring in sufficient mechanisms for objectivity and this exercise can be carried out mechanically by using a suitable computer and software. Determination of correct Prakruti is vital since further inventions and therapeutics are based on that consideration[23].

According to Ayurveda every material either organic or inorganic has certain attributes. Ayurveda has illustrated twenty such attributes or Gunas. These attributes have a definite effect on TriDoshas and then on the Panchamahabhootas. Thus, one can selectively use variety of combinations of materials to achieve a desired, pre-determined impact to bring an imbalance TriDoshas

[23] Svoboda R. Prakruti - Your Ayurvedic Constitution (1996), Motilal Banarasidas Publishers Private limited. New Delhi-110007, India.

into equilibrium. The Ayurvedic pharmacology and therapeutics are based on the actions and counteractions of selectively used materials with predetermined combination of these attributes for desired balance of TriDoshas. Another important feature of Ayurvedic pharmacology is its depth in understanding effects of these materials after they enter in the human body and the effects thereof on the three humors KPV. This Ayurvedic Pharmacokinetics and Pharmacodynamics is vital in therapeutics and dietetics. Ayurveda has described six tastes as identified by tongue or Rasa: Sweet, Sour, Salty, Pungent, Bitter and Astringent. These substances will produce two types of effects (Hot or Cold) during the digestive phase, which is called as Virya. The same material will produce post-digestive effects of sweet, sour or pungent type, which is called as Vipaka. Generally it is observed that sweet and salty tastes will have sweet Vipaka; Sour taste has sour and pungent, bitter, astringent have pungent Vipaka. Rasa, Virya and Vipaka directly influence the TriDosha, Nutrition and Tissue development of SaptaDhatu: Rasa (plasma), Rakta (blood), Mansa (Muscle), Meda (Adipose), Asthi (Bones), Majja (Nerves) and Shukra (semen). Exhaustive information is available in Ayurvedic literature that can be converted into a large database giving information of various foods[24], herbs, medicines and other materials with their taste, actions and utility in different disorders. An innovative method to help quantitative representations of various Ayurvedic concepts including Prakruti, Rasa, Guna and such has been developed by Indian Institute of Chemical Technology. This technology has been registered as Herboprint and is patented. Herboprint

---

[24] The Ayurvedic Cookbook. Amadea Moringstar, (1990), Lotus Press, Santa Fe.

essentially gives a three dimentional HPLC fingerprint with Ayurvedic property profile[25].

It would be extremely valuable to develop an Ayurvedic database available in classic texts. First, it could be used for bio-prospecting to identify potential new sources of medicines. Second, it could give information about likely effects of Ayurvedic treatments ranging from primary taste to post digestive effects. Third, it could give information about safety and efficacy along with possible indications and contraindications. Fourth, it could give information on therapeutic potential and selective benefits to people with different constitutions. Most importantly, it would greatly facilitate intentional, focused and safe natural product drug discovery and development.

❐❐❐

[25] Vijay Kumar, Herboprint- A novel method of analysis 2002, IICT, Hyderabad.

3 Natural Product and Drug Discovery

The R&D thrust in the pharmaceutical sector is focused on development of new drugs, innovative/indigenous processes for known drugs and development of plant based drugs through investigation of leads from the traditional systems of medicine. In addition, many nutraceuticals are being consumed from unregulated markets for their perceived benefits in health care and improvement of quality of life.

Natural pharmaceuticals, nutraceuticals and cosmeceuticals are of great importance as a reservoir of chemical diversity aimed at new drug discovery and can be explored as potential antimicrobial, cardiovascular, immunosuppressive, and anticancer drugs. Around 80% of all such products are of plant origin; their sales exceeded $ 65 billion in 2003. Examples of plant products and derivatives used by the pharmaceutical industry include Paclitaxel, Vincristine, Vinblastine, Artemisinin, Camptothecin, Podophyllotoxin and such.

The nutraceutical marketplace in Europe is estimated to be $ 9 billion, while the US marketplace, estimated to be $10-12 billion in 2003, is expanding at a compounded rate of more than 20% per year. US Congress has fueled the rapid growth of nutraceuticals with the passage of the Dietary Supplement Health and Education Act (DSHEA) in 1994. Globally, there have been efforts to monitor quality and regulate the growing business of herbal drugs and traditional medicine.

Introduction

Natural products including plants, animals and minerals have been the basis of treatment of human diseases. Modern medicine or allopathy has gradually developed over the years of scientific and observational efforts of scientists – however, the basis of its development remains in the roots of traditional medicine and therapies. The history of medicine includes many ludicrous therapies. Nevertheless, the ancient wisdom has been the basis of modern medicine and will remain as one important source of future medicine and therapeutics. Even during the early part of this century, plants were a vital source of raw material for medicines. The future of natural product drug discovery will be more holistic, personalized and involve wise use of ancient and modern therapeutic skills in complementary manner so that maximum benefits can be given to patients and the community.[26]

Greek physician Galen (129-200 AD) devised the first Pharmacopoeia describing the appearance, properties and use of many plants of his time. The foundations of modern pharmaceutical industry were laid when techniques were developed to produce synthetic replacements for many of the medicines that had been derived from the forest. Natural Product Chemistry actually began with the work of Serturner who first isolated morphine from opium. This in-turn was obtained from opium poppy (*Papaver somniferum*)

[26] Patwardhan Bhushan, Ayurveda and Future Drug Development, International Journal of Alternative and Complementary Medicine 1992, 10(12), 9-11.

by processes that have been used for over 5000 years. Many such similar developments followed. Quinine from Cinchona tree had its origin in the royal households of South American Incas. Before the first European explorers arrived, the native people of the Americas had developed complex medical systems complete with diagnosis and treatment of physical as well as spiritual illnesses. Indigenous peoples derived medicines and poisons from thousands of plants. Review of some of the plants that originated from Central and South America indicate that most of them either had potentially toxic or poisonous characters or were from food sources. Following are few examples[27]: In the early 1500's, Indian fever bark was one of the first medicinal plants to find appreciative consumers in Europe. Taken from the cinchona tree (*Cinchona officinalis*), the bark was used as an infusion by native people of the Andes and Amazon highlands to treat fevers. Jesuit missionaries brought the bark back to Europe. By the early sixteenth century, this medicine had grown in popularity and was known as "Jesuit fever bark". The name coca (*Erythroxylum coca*) comes from an Aymara word meaning simply "tree". In Andean cultures, the leaves of the coca tree have been primarily chewed to obtain the benefits. From ancient times, indigenous people have added an alkaline such as crushed seashells or burnt plant ashes to leaves in order to activate the pharmacologically part of coca. In 1860, a German chemist isolated the chemical responsible for the plant's power, now known as cocaine. Carl Koler found cocaine could act as a local anesthetic in eye surgery. As the years passed, scientists found that cocaine paralyzed nerve endings responsible for transmitting pain. As a local anesthetic, it revolutionized several surgical and dental procedures. Pot curare Arrow head poison used in the East

[27] Steven King, Medicines that changed the world, Pacific Discovery, 1992: 45(1), 23-31.

Amazon is predominately from the species *Strychnos guianensis*. Tube curare in the West Amazon is from *Chrondrodendron tomentosum* from which the curare in modern medicine is made from and named as tubocurarine. The jaborandi tree (*Pilocarpus jaborandi*) secretes alkaloid-rich oil. Several substances are extracted from this aromatic oil, including the alkaloid pilocarpine, a weapon against the blinding disease glaucoma. American Indians used pineapple (*Ananas comosos)* poultices to reduce inflammation in wounds and other skin injuries, to aid digestion and to cure stomachache on the island of Guadeloupe. In 1891 an enzyme that broke down proteins (bromelain) was isolated from the fresh juice of pineapple was found to break down blood clots. Even now, many pharmaceuticals have their origin in botanicals. Just few more to mention include Atropine, Hyoscine, Digoxin, Cholchicine, Emetine, and like. Reserpine is an anti-hypertensive alkaloid (*Rauwolfia serpentina*) that became available as a result of work carried out by Ciba in India. It is pertinent to note that most of these early discoveries are based on potentially poisonous sources based on little traditions.

Discovering Medicines or Poisons?

One of the major problems with traditional indigenous medicine is discovering a reliable 'living tradition' rather than relying upon second hand accounts of their value and use. In many parts of the world the indigenous system of medicine have almost completely broken down and disappeared. This includes mostly developed countries and some developing countries where the indigenous population is marginalized. In others, the system is fragmented with the use of indigenous materials being limited to small tribal and geographical areas, which is the case in many parts of Africa. Although, the little traditions might have excellent knowledge about medicinal and poisonous properties of botanicals, thus far, researchers have mainly focused on poisonous sources. First, it is relatively easy to present and demonstrate poisonous characteristics of botanicals. Second, there may not be a written documentation, so the word—of-mouth poisonous characters get attention. Third, for an outsider, poisonous characteristics differentiate in between ordinary and extra-ordinary material for pharmaceutical development. Fourth, a considerable time period is required to demonstrate true medicinal activities with proven safety profile. To counter this focus on the potentially harmful portions of traditional medicines, great traditions must work from their relatively organized database, so that the botanical material that is available can be tested using modern scientific methods. Ayurveda and Chinese Medical systems thus have an important role in bio-prospecting of new medicines.

Serendipity and Synthetic Dominance

Pharmaceutical research took a major leap when alongside natural product chemistry, pharmacologists, microbiologists and biochemists began to unravel the chemistry of natural processes in human, animals, plants and microorganisms. Advances in organic synthetic chemistry led to identification of many key chemical molecules, which offered more opportunities to develop novel compounds. Many new drugs emerged by this route, particularly those now used to treat infections, infestations, cancers, ulcers, heart and blood pressure conditions. Many drugs were developed through random screening of thousands of chemicals while others came in a serendipity arising from sharp-eyed observations of physicians and scientists. Examples of such drugs include Sulfonamides, Isoniazid, Anti-psychotic, Anti-histaminic and Penicillin. Emergence of the modern pharmaceutical industry is an outcome of all these different activities that developed potent single molecules with highly selective activity for a wide variety of different conditions. The drugs produced in many cases improved on nature, such as with the local anesthetics from cocaine, which avoided its dangerous effects on blood pressure and chloroquine, which is much less toxic than quinine. These successes and many more like them resulted in reduced interest in natural product drug discovery and many major drug companies neglected such divisions. Work on developing new drugs for the treatment of the world's major diseases, Malaria, Trypanosomiasis, Filariasis, Tuberculosis, Schistosomiasis, Leshmaniasis, Amoebiasis came almost to a stand still. In addition, although botanical medicines continued to be produced in every country, the clinical efficacy of these medicines was usually not evaluated and the composition of these complex mixtures was only crudely analyzed. Thus, herbal medicines became the domain of 'old wives tales' and quack medicine, and many believed that they were only used for the exploitation of the sick, desperate, and gullible. Sadly, those herbal medicines that were tested continued to be poor in quality control both for materials and clinical efficacy.

Back to Traditional Wisdom

Lag phase for botanical medicine is now rapidly changing for a number of reasons. First, problems with drug resistant microorganisms, side effects of modern drugs, and emerging diseases where no medicines are available, have encouraged an interest in plants once again as a significant source of new medicines. Second, pharmaceutical scientists are getting short of new lead structures since they have exhausted most known ones. Third, there have been several impressive successes with botanical medicines, such as Quinghaosu and Artemisinin from Chinese medicine.

Considerable research on pharmacognosy, chemistry, pharmacology and clinical therapeutics has been carried out on Ayurvedic medicinal plants[28]. A large numbers of molecules have come out of Ayurvedic experiential base include Rauwolfia alkaloids for hypertension, Psoralens in Vitiligo, Holarrhena alkaloids in Amoebiasis, Guggulsterons as hypolipidemic agents, Mucuna pruriens for Parkinson's disease, Piperidines as bioavailability enhancers, Baccosides in mental retention, Picrosides in hepatic protection, Phyllanthins as antivirals, Curcumines in inflammation, Withanolides, and many other steroidal lactones and glycosides as immunomodulators[29]. Forth, a number of synthetic drugs have adverse and unacceptable side effects. Fifth, a whole range of chronic and difficult to treat diseases such as cancers, cardiovascular disease, diabetes, rheumatism and newer diseases like AIDS all require new effective drugs. Sixth, most of the population of developing countries have relied and will continue to rely on traditional natural medicines for variety of reasons including high costs of modern medicines.

Research, Development and Markets

Even now, about thirty percent of the worldwide sales of drugs are based on natural products. Although recombinant proteins and peptides account for increasing sales rates, the superiority of low-molecular mass compounds in human therapy remains undisputed mainly due to more favorable compliance and bioavailability properties. Approaches to improve and accelerate the joint drug discovery and development process are expected to take place mainly from innovation in drug target elucidation

---

[28] Dahanukar S.A., Kulkarni R.A., Rege N.N. Pharmacology of medicinal plants and natural products. Indian Journal of Pharmacology 2000; 32: S81-S118.

[29] Patwardhan Bhushan. Ayurvedaa: The Designer Medicine. Indian Drugs 2000; 37(5): 213-227.

and lead structure discovery. The need for new concepts to generate large compound collection with improved structural diversity has been correctly emphasized[30]. Commercially, plant-derived medicines are worth about $14 billion a year in the United States and $40 billion worldwide. Americans paid an estimated $21.2 billion for services provided by alternative medicine practitioners[31]. A 1997 survey estimated that over 12% of adults had used herbal medicine during 1996 as compared with 2.5% in 1990, resulting in a business of $5.1 billion[32]. In 1985, Lilly Research Laboratories sold roughly $100 million worth of Vincristine and Vinblastine — the periwinkle derivatives used to treat childhood leukemia and Hodgkin's disease — and turned a stunning 8 percent profit. In the early 1990s, the U.S. National Cancer Institute earmarked $8 million to screen 50,000 natural substances for activity against 100 cancer cell lines and the AIDS virus. China, Germany, India, and Japan, among others, are also screening wild species for new drugs.

Plant-derived drugs have an important place in both traditional and modern medicine. For this reason a special effort to maintain the great diversity of plant species would undoubtedly help to alleviate human suffering in the long term. Proven agro-industrial technologies need to be applied to the cultivation and processing of medicinal plants and the manufacture of herbal medicines[33]. The mass screening of plants in the search for new drugs is vastly expensive

---

[30] Grabley S; Thiericke R, Bioactive agents from natural sources: trends in discovery and application. Adv Biochem Eng Biotechnol 1999;64:101-54.

[31] Eisenberg D.M. et. Al, Trends in alternative medicine use in US, The Journal of the American Medical Association, 1998 November 11.

[32] De Smet, Herbal Remedies, The New England Journal of Medicine, 2002: 347: 2046-2056.

[33] Akerele O. Nature's medicinal bounty: don't throw it away. W.H.O. Geneva, Switzerland. World Health Forum 1993; 14(4): 390-5.

and inefficient. It would be cheaper and perhaps more productive to re-examine plant remedies described in ancient and mediaeval texts[34]. Botanicals have always been a major source of medicine for humankind and early references were often guides to the medicinal plants of a particular region. Even today, approximately one quarter of all prescription pharmaceuticals contain at least one plant-derived ingredient. For example, Atropa belladonna, the source of atropine, is from G. Pabst's 1887 atlas of the medicinal plants of Europe entitled Kohler's Medizinal Pflanzen. Botanists from the Missouri Botanical Garden have been working with pharmaceutical researchers in the search for new medicines for more than ten years and have collected more than 25,000 samples for screening. Many higher plants produce economically important organic compounds such as oils, resins, tannins, natural rubber, gums, waxes, dyes, flavors, fragrances, pharmaceuticals, and pesticides. However, most species of higher plants have never been described, much less surveyed for chemical or biologically active constituents, and new sources of commercially valuable materials remain to be discovered. Advances in biotechnology, particularly methods for culturing plant cells and tissues, should provide new means for the commercial processing of even rare plants and the chemicals they produce. These new technologies will extend and enhance the usefulness of plants as renewable resources of valuable chemicals. In the future, biologically active plant-derived chemicals can be expected to play an increasingly significant role in the commercial development

---

[34] Holland BK. Prospecting for drugs in ancient texts. Nature 1994 Jun 30; 369 (6483), Comment in Nature 1994 Sep 1; 371 (6492): 9, Comment in: Nature 1994 Nov 10; 372 (6502): 124; Comment in: Nature 1995 Aug 17; 376 (6541): 546; Cox PA. The ethnobotanical approach to drug discovery. Scientific American 1994 Jun; 270(6): 82.

of new products for regulating plant growth and for insect and weed control[35].

Some of the prominent commercial plant derived medicinal compounds include: Colchicum, Colchicine, betulinic acid, Camptothecin, topotecan (Hycamtin®), CPT-11 (irinotecan, Camptosar®), 9-aminocamptothecin, delta-9-tetrahydrocannabinol (dronabinol, Marinol®), beta lapachone, lapachol, Podophyllotoxin, etoposide, podophyllinic acid, vinblastine (Velban®), vincristine (leurocristine, Oncovin®), vindesine (Eldisine®, Fildesin®), vinorelbine (Navelbine®), docetaxel (Taxotere®), paclitaxel (Taxol®), Tubocurarine, Pilocarpine, Scopolamine.

The possibility for developing new drugs from rain forest resources reflects how successful plant-derived drugs can be. All 119 plant-derived drugs used worldwide in 1991 came from fewer than 90 of the 250,000 plant species that have been identified. Each of such medicinal plants is a unique chemical factory, asmentioned by Norman Farnsworth of the University of Illinois at Chicago, that are capable of synthesizing unlimited numbers of highly complex and unusual chemical substances whose structures could otherwise escape the imagination. The ultimate goal of ethnopharmacology should be to identify drugs to alleviate human illness *via* a thorough analysis of plants alleged to be useful in human cultures throughout the world[36].

---

[35] Balandrin MF; Klocke JA; Wurtele ES; Bollinger WH. Natural plant chemicals: sources of industrial and medicinal materials. Science 1985 Jun 7; 228(4704): 1154-60]; Bonati A,. Medicinal plants and industry. J. Ethnopharmacol 1980 Jun; 2(2): 167-71; Wijesekera RO. Is there an industrial future for phytopharmaceutical drugs? An outline of UNIDO programs in the sector. Chemical Industries Branch, United Nations Industrial Development Organization. J Ethnopharmacol 1991 Apr; 32(1-3): 217-24.

[36] The role of Ethnopharmacology in drug development. Farnsworth NR, Ciba Found Symp 1990;154:2-11; discussion 11-21; Ethnopharmacology and Western medicine. Phillipson JD; Anderson, Journal of Ethnopharmacology 1989;25(1):61-72.

Great Traditions – Key to discovery

Many of the major pharmaceutical corporations have renewed their strategies in favor of natural product drug discovery. However, the 'Discovery Engines' that are largely used are still based on the knowledge and information obtained from 'little traditions' and is based on comparatively short-duration experiences. (What are "discovery enginesAlthough there is a re-generation of natural product drug research, still the real 'great traditions' remain under-explored and they are really the true sources of future medicines.

Natural product research continues to explore variety of lead structures, which may be used as templates for the development of new drugs by the pharmaceutical industry. While microbial products have been the mainstay of industrial natural products discovery, in recent years phytochemistry has again become a field of active interest. Drug discovery programs based on microbial products and phytochemicals are discussed and contrasted[37]. To take a few examples, Glaxo PLC most recently has pursued this interest by use of such materials as templates for new lead discovery through the expertise and facilities in its Natural Products Discovery Department. Extracts and fermentation broths are screened in order to detect bioactive principles[38]. Many other multinationals and academic institutions have created joint research programs for plant medicine research, such as Searle, University of Ghana and BioResources, Virginia Polytechnic Institute, Bedrijf Geneesmiddelen Voorziening Suriname (BGVS), Conservation International-

---

[37] Borris J Natural products research: perspectives from a major pharmaceutical company, , Merck Research Laboratories, J Ethnopharmacol 1996 Apr;51 (1-3):29.

[38] Turner D. J Natural product source material use in the pharmaceutical industry: the Glaxo experience. Ethnopharmacol 1996 Apr;51(1-3):39-43.

Suriname, and Bristol-Myers Squibb Pharmaceutical Research Institute. The National Institutes of Health, the National Science Foundation, and USAID sponsor some of such projects. University of Chicago at Illinois, University of Mississippi, Xeenova, Shaman Pharmaceuticals, Ayur-Core, Inc and Bio-Ved Pharmaceuticals are few more examples. Many traditional Ayurveda and Indian pharmaceutical companies have changed in favor of science-based research. Dabur, Zandu, Arya Vaidya Shala, Nicholas Piramal, Lupin, Ranbaxy, are few prominent examples. The Pharmaceutical Research and Development Committee (PDRC) Report of Ministry of Chemicals, Government of India also underlines importance of traditional knowledge[39].

From the point of view of drug researches, there are many factors that encourage them to pursue research in natural products. First, unmet therapeutic needs; second, the remarkable diversity of both chemical structures and biological activities of naturally occurring secondary metabolites; third, the utility of bioactive natural products as biochemical and molecular probes, fourth, the development of novel and sensitive techniques to detect biologically active natural products; fifth, improved techniques to isolate, purify, and structurally characterize these active constituents, and last, advances in solving the demand for supply of complex natural products. Opportunities for multidisciplinary research that joins the forces of natural products chemistry, molecular and cellular biology, synthetic and analytical chemistry, biochemistry, and pharmacology to exploit the vast diversity of chemical structures and biological activities of natural products are

---

[39] Mashelkar R.A. Transforming India into the Knowledge Power, PDRC Report, Government of India, November 1999.

best discussed by Clark[40]. The exploration of structural chemical databases comprising a wide variety of chemotypes, in conjunction with databases on target genes and proteins, will facilitate the creation of new chemical entities through computational molecular modeling for pharmacological evaluation[41].

In the natural product drug discovery it is important to follow a system-theory and systems biology applications to facilitate the process[42]. Routine random efforts are not likely to increase the desired success rate of discovery. Taking example of National Cancer Institute (NCI) efforts, between 1960 and 1981 they screened 114,000 extracts of 35,000 plants, mainly collected in temperate regions. Of the three clinically active anticancer drugs so far discovered in that program, none was isolated from a plant collected on an ethnobotanical basis, though various Taxus species as the sources of Taxol are reported for medicinal use. Since 1986, the NCI has focused its collections in tropical and subtropical regions worldwide; collections cover a broad taxonomic range, though priority is given to medicinal plants when relevant information is available. As of August 1993, 21,881 extracts derived from over 10,500 samples had been tested in a screen for activity against the human immunodeficiency virus (HIV); 2320 of these extracts were of medicinal plant origin. Approximately 18% of both the total number of extracts and the medicinal plant-derived extracts

---

[40] Clark AM Natural products as a resource for new drugs. University of Mississippi, Pharm Res 1996 Aug;13(8):1133-44.

[41] Nisbet LJ; Moore M. Will natural products remain an important source of drug research for the future?. Curr Opin Biotechnol 1997 Dec;8(6):708-12; Biodiversity prospecting and benefit-sharing: perspectives from the field. Soejarto DD, J. Ethnopharmacol 1996 Apr;51(1-3):1-15.

[42] Leroy Hood, Principles, Practice and Future of Systems Biology, Drug Discovery Today 2003: 8(10); 436-438.

showed significant anti-HIV activity; in each instance about 90% of the active extracts were aqueous. The activity of the aqueous extracts has been attributed mainly to the presence of polysaccharides or tannins. Four plant- derived compounds are in pre-clinical development at the NCI; only one of the four sources plants, obtained from a non-contract source, was collected on an ethnobotanical basis. At this stage the results indicate that the modified NCI collection policy offered the better chances for the discovery and development of agents for the treatment of AIDS and cancer[43].

By integrating the sciences of ethnobotany, medicine and plant natural product chemistry, it is possible to achieve time and cost savings for the identification of active compounds and pre-clinical development of its initial products. Numerous drugs have entered the international pharmacopoeia *via* the study of ethnobotany and traditional medicine[44]. It is from this knowledge that future considerations of ethnopharmacology need to be determined. In view of the progress of western medicine, not only new synthetic drugs but botanical drugs also will have to fulfill the international requirements on quality, safety and efficacy[45].

---

[43] Cragg GM; Boyd MR; Cardellina JH 2nd; Newman DJ; Snader KM; McCloud. Ethnobotany and drug discovery: the experience of the US National Cancer Institute Developmental Therapeutics Program, National Cancer Institute, Bethesda, Ciba Foundation Symposium 1994;185:178-90; 190-96. Kitagawa I, Elucidation of scientific basis for traditional medicines and exploitation of new naturally occurring drugs, Yakugaku Zasshi 1992 Jan 112:1 1-41.

[44] De Smet PA, The role of plant-derived drugs and herbal medicines in healthcare. Pharmaceutical Care Unit, Drugs 1997 Dec; 54(6): 801-40; King SR; Tempesta MS. From shaman to human clinical trials: the role of industry in ethnobotany, conservation and community reciprocity. Ciba Found Symp 1994; 185:197-206; discussion 206-13.

[45] Vogel HG. Similarities between various systems of traditional medicine: Considerations for the future of ethnopharmacology, J. Ethnopharmacol 1991 Dec 35:2 179-90.

The origin of all such knowledge in India is in the Great Tradition of Ayurveda, which is a living tradition in practice even today. Indian health care consists of medical pluralism and Ayurveda still remains dominating even as compared to the modern medicine particularly for treatments of variety of chronic disease conditions[46]. India has about 45,000 plant species and medicinal properties have been assigned to several thousand. About 2000 figure frequently in the literature; indigenous systems commonly employ about 500. Some recent work in drug development relates to species of Commiphora (used as a hypolipidaemic agent), Picrorhiza (which is hepatoprotective), Bacopa (memory enhancer), Curcuma (anti-inflammatory) and Asclepias (cardiotonic)[47].

Review of Top Ten Ayurvedic Drugs

Charak Samhita is one of the most cited Ayurvedic classic books that we have referred to select Top 20 Ayurvedic Drugs. To augment this effort we have short-listed some broad Reviews[48,49] Database[50] and Compendium[51] generally covering research on most of the

---

[46] Waxler-Morrison NE. Plural medicine in India & Sri Lanka: do Ayurvedic and Western medical practices differ? Social Science and Medicine 1988 27:5 531-44.

[47] Jain SK, Ethnobotany and research on medicinal plants in India, Ciba Found Symp 1994;185:153-64; discussion 164-8.

[48] Dahanukar S.A, Kulkarni R.A, Rege N.N., Pharmacology of Medicinal Plants. Indian Journal of Pharmacology 2000; 32:S; 81-118.

[49] T.P.A Devasagayam and K.B. Sainis. Immune system and antioxidants: especially those derived from Indian Medicinal plants. Indian Journal of Experimental Biology Vol. 40, June 2002,639-655.

[50] Sharma P.C, Yelne M.B and Dennis T.J (2001). Database on Medicinal Plants used in Ayurveda (Volume 1-3). Published by Central Council for Research in Ayurveda and Siddha, New Delhi - 110058.

[51] Rastogi Ram P. and Mehrotra B.N (1998). Compendium of Indian Medicinal Plants. Joint Publication of Central Drug Research Institute, Lucknow and National Institute of Science Communication and Information Resources (Vol 1-6), New Delhi -110012.

popular Ayurvedic drugs. We have used Medline search number of hits as an indicator. Search after giving the Ayurvedic name resulted in much smaller number of hits as compared to their respective botanical names. This is mainly because similar botanicals are used and researched in different parts of the world. One more reason for this as in case of Curcuma is because of its popular name turmeric and the Ayurvedic name is rarely used. Some of the Ayurvedic drugs when searched for Sanskrit names did not give any hits, which indicate potential researchable areas. In some cases such as *Phyllanthus embelica* (earlier known as *Emblica officinalis*), the number of hits is less than anticipated because of recent change in its botanical name. For some drugs such as Ricinus (source of caster oil) maximum hits were obtained but most of the research is related to industrial use and not medicinal. Ashwagandha remained most researched plant drug from this list. For the purpose of present review, we have short listed the Top 10 Ayurvedic drugs (randomly organized) to summarize their properties and uses along with key references.

Shunthi/Ginger (*Zingiber officinale*)

Zingiber officinale (Ginger) has been commonly used in household medicines for ages. It is also known as Mahaaushadi meaning 'a great medicine.' It is used for coughs, bronchitis and as a stomach tonic. A rapid and accurate HPTLC method for detection, monitoring and quantitation of ginger from Ayurvedic preparations has been devised[52]. Cancer chemotherapy causes severe nausea, vomitting and abdominal discomfort which limits therapy. Anticancer drugs like Cisplatin causes nausea, vomitting and inhibition of gastric emptying. The antiemetic effect of

---

[52] Sane R.T. *et al.*, A HPTLC Method for the quantitative analysis of ginger from an Ayuvedic preparation, Indian Drugs 33(9) 462-464.

the acetone and ethanolic extract of ginger against cisplatin-induced emesis in drugs was evaluated. Significant reversal of cisplatin-induced delay in gastric emptying was seen. Therefore, ginger as an antiemetic for cancer chemotherapy may also be useful in improving gastrointestinal side effects associated with cancer chemotherapy. The antiemetic effect of ginger may be due to the scavenging activity of gingerol. Another study showed that the 5 HT 3 - receptor-blocking activity could also be the reason for the antiemetic effect. They concluded that ginger is worth further clinical evaluation as an antiemetic against cisplatin induced emesis[53]. Another study involved use of Pyrogallol, a free radical generator that has been shown to cause a significant delay in gastric emptying in rats that mimics the pathogenesis of gastrointestinal illnesses in which free radicals are involved. In the study the inhibitory effect of Pyrogallol on gastric emptying was dose dependently reversed by ginger acetone extract and the effect was significant at doses of 250 and 500 mg/ kg.

In addition, the antioxidant activity of ginger has been extensively studied[54]. The free radical scavenging and /or the antiserotonergic action of ginger could be mechanism to reverse pyrogallol-induced delay in gastric emptying. The combination of the ginger acetone extract along with the antioxidants Vitamin C and Vitamin E produced a significant reverse as compared to ginger acetone extract alone. Thus there are beneficial effects of the ginger extract in improving symptoms such as abdominal discomfort and bloating[55].

---

[53] Sharma S.S, *et al.* Antiemetic efficacy of ginger against Cisplatin induced emesis in dogs, Journal of Ethnopharmacology, 57(1997) 93-96.

[54] Shobhana S and Naidu K.A., Antioxidant activity of selected Indian spices., Prostaglandins Leukot Essent Fatty Acids 2000 62:2 107-10.

[55] Gupta Y.K. and Sharma M. Reversal of Pyrogallol induced dealy in gastric emptying in rats by ginger, Methods Find Exp Clin Pharmacol 2001, 23(9), 501-503.

Guduchi (*Tinospora cordifolia*)

Tinospora cordifolia is a plant belonging to the Rasayana group of Charaka Samhita whichgiven for prevention of diseases and strengthening of both physical and mental health. It has been extensively studied for its immunostimulant activity. Chronic liver damage in humans and experimental animals is characterized by deposition of fibrous tissues in the liver. Kupffer cells are considered as a major determinant in the outcome of liver injury. This activity was studied in a model of chronic liver disease. The effect of *Tinospora cordifolia* on Kupffer cell function was studied using carbon clearance test as a parameter in rats. A significant improvement in kupffer cell function was seen and a trend towards normalization was observed[56]. Immunomodulatory activity was studied and colony-forming units of the granulocyte-macrophage series (CFU-GM) activity was measured in serum of mice treated with Tinospora. Treatment resulted in leucocytosis with predominant neutrophilia. There was significant increase in CFU-GM activity in the serum. This haemopoeitic growth factor leads to an array of effects including induction of leucocytosis as well as prevention of cytotoxic chemotherapy induced neutropenia indicated its great potential as an immunomodulator[57]. The complications observed in obstructive jaundice are secondary to endotoxicaemia. A study was undertaken to evaluate the effects of *Tinospora cordifolia* in a rat model of cholestasis. Results showed reduced endotoxicaemia after tinospora cordifolia therapy. The Phase I clinical study carried out

---

[56] Deepa. S. Nagarkalli,. Rege N. N,.Desai N.K, Dahanukar S.A . Modulation of Kupffer cell activity by Tinospora cordifolia in liver damage, Journal of Postgraduate Medicine 1994: 40 (2).

[57] Thatte U.M.,.Rao S.G.A,.Dahanukar S.A, Tinospora cordifolia induces colony stimulating activity in serum., Journal of Postgraduate Medicine 199140(4), 202-203.

on healthy volunteers to evaluate safety did not reveal any alterations in biochemical, immunological or radiological parameters. Maximum clinical exploration was done in patients with obstructive jaundice. Tinospora was used as an add-on regime to conventional therapy. This was associated with decrease in septicaemia. It was also found to potentiate neutrophil activity. The neutrophils of these patients also showed an increase in phagocytic activity, which manifested as a feeling of well being, and improved appetite. No side effects were observed with *Tinospora cordifolia*[58].

Shatavari (*Asparagus racemosus*)

The possible antioxidant effects of crude extract and a purified fraction of *Asparagus racemosus* against membrane damage induced by the free radicals generated during gamma-radication were examined in rat liver mitochondria. The extracts have potent antioxidant properties *in vitro* in mitochondrial membranes of rat liver. They also protected superoxide dismutase and protein thiols from inactivation. This contributes to the cellular antioxidant defense system[59]. The hypothesis that macrophages appear to play a pivotal role in the development of intraperitoneal adhesions, modulation of macrophage activity, therefore is likely to provide a tool for prevention of adhesions. The effect of *Asparagus racemosus,* an immuno stimulant drug, was evaluated in albino rats with intraperitoneal adhesions induced by caecal rubbing. After treatment with *Asparagus Racemosus,* a significant decrease was observed in the

---

[58] Rege N.N., Javle H, Bapat R.D., Dahanukar S.A. Antiendotoxic effect of Tinospora cordifolia; an experimental study in rats, Indian Journal of Pharmaceutical Sciences 1998: 60(5) 6.

[59] Kamath Jayashree, A. Devasagayam P.A, Venkatachalam S.R. Antioxidant properties of Asparagus Racemosus against damage induced by gama-radiation in rat liver mitochondria, Journal of Ethnopharmacology,(2000: 71; 425-435.

adhesion scores. There was also a significant increase in activity of macrophages. This study shows how *Asparagus Racemosus* help in the prevention and management of post-operative adhesions[60].

Nimba/Neem (*Azadirachta indica*)

This herbal treatment is commonly known as Neem tree. Various extracts were studied for castor oil induced diarrhea; gastrointestinal motility and prostaglandin E2 induced enteropooling. Results of the study suggest the prostaglandin inhibition is the primary outcome and mild inhibition of gastrointestinal motility as a secondary effect[61]. The ethanolic extract was studied for carbon tetrachloride induced hepatic changes in albino rats. The changes were assessed by serum enzyme profile that include glutamic oxaloacetate transaminase (GOT), glutamic pyruvic transaminase (GPT), alkalline phosphatase (AP), bilirubin(B) and hepatic triglycerides (HTG) levels, histological changes in liver and pentobarbitone sleeping time as a functional parameter. There was significant reversal of biochemical, histological and functional changes induced by carbon tetrachloride in rats by ethanol extract treatment[62]. Early epithelialisation with acceptable scar and maintenance and function of the concerned part are important goals in burn care. A study was carried out to evaluate tolerability and efficacy of a topical formulation of *Azadirachta indica* in patients with burns. The formulation

---

[60] Rege Nirmala.N., Nazareth H.M., Ann Isaac,.Karandikar S.M,.Dahanukar Sharadini. Immunotherapeutic modulation of Introperitoneal Adhesions of Asparagus racemosus. Journal of Postgraduate Medicine 1989: 35(4) 199-203.

[61] Mujumdar A.M., Antidiarrhoeal activity of Azadirachta indica leaf extract., Indian Drugs 35(7) 417-4120, 1998.

[62] Mujumdar A.M., Upadhye A.S.and.Pradhan A.M, Effect of Azadirachta indica leaf extract in carbontetrachloride induced hepatic damage in albino rats, Ind J of Pharm Sci. 199860(6), 363-367.

showed positive results comparable with Silver Sulphadiazine. Azadirachta indica was reported to be safe and effective prohealer for burns, which lead to a better cosmetic outcome[63].

Ashwagandha (*Withania somnifera*)

Ashwagandha is relatively well-studied plant. Chemopreventive activity was shown in experimentally induced fibro sarcoma tumors. Ashwagandha significantly reduced the tumor incidence, tumor volume and enhanced the survival of the mice. Liver biochemical parameters revealed a significant modulated (do you mean modulator?) of reduced glutathione, lipid peroxidases, glutathione-s-transferase, catalase, and superoxide dismutase in extract treateed mice. The mechanism of chemopreventive activity of *Withania somnifera* extract may be due to its antioxidant and detoxifying properties[64]. Effect of pre- and co- treatment of hydroalcoholic root extract of *Withania somnifera* at different doses was investigated against Isoproterenol-induced myocardial infarction in rats. At dose of 100 mg/kg there was maximum cardioprotective effect. Results were confirmed by histopathological findings[65]. Ashwagandha was compared with Ginseng for adaptogenic and antistress activity and was found to be a better drug of choice with additional anti-inflammatory

---

[63] Rege N.N, Dahanukar S.A, Ginde V, Thatte U.M, Bapat R.D., safety and efficacy of Azadirachta indica in patients with second degree burns, The Indian Practitioner, Vol 52, No 4, 240-240, April 1999.

[64] Prakash Jai, Gupta S.K, Kochupillai V., Singh N, Gupta Y.K and Joshi S. Chemopreventive Activity of Withania somnifera in experimentally induced Fibrosarcoma tumooours in swiss Albino mice, Phytother. Res.2001: 15, 240-244.

[65] Sharma Meenu, Kishore Kamal, Suresh, Gupta K,. Joshi S, Arya D.S. Withania somnifera provides cardiac protection in Isoproterenol induced myocardial infarction, Intl J Med Biol Environ 2000: 26(2), 213-220.

activity[66]. Immunomodulatory activity has also been demonstrated in experimental immuneinflammation and cyclophosphamide induced myelo-suppression[67].

Pippali (*Piper longum*)

The ethanolic extract of *Piper longum* fruit was tested for cytotoxicity using the brine shrimp lethality test. It showed potent cytotoxic activity[68]. Piperine is a constituent of various spices that are used as common food additives. The reproductive toxicity of piperine was studied in albino mice. Piperine increased the period of diestrous phase, which seemed to result in decreased mating performance and fertility. Prostaglandin E-1 induced acute inflammation of rat paw was significantly reduced after piperine treatment. Thus piperine was shown to interfere with several crucial reproductive events in mammalian model[69]. A reverse phase HPLC method to determine pierine in different medicinally used Piperine samples has been developed. The method is precise, sensitive, reproducible and easy to perform. The sensitivity of the method was 0.1mcg and the linearity was observed in the range of 0.1 mcg to 0.8 mcg. This method can be used for the detection and monitoring of Piperine[70]. A spectrophotometric method has been

---

[66] Grandhi A. Mujumdar A, Patwardhan B. Comparative pharmacology of Ashwagandha and Ginseng. Journal of Ethnopharmacology, 1994, 44, 131-135.

[67] Agarwal Ramesh, Diwanay S, Patki P., Patwardhan B. Studies on immunomodulatory activity of Ashwagandha in experimental immune inflammation. Journal of Ethnopharmacology 1999, 67, 27-35.

[68] Padmaja R., Arun P.C, .Prashanth D,. Deepak M, .Amit A,.Anjana M., Brine shrimp lethality bioassay of selected Indian Medicinal plants, Fitoterapia 73(2002) 508-510.

[69] Daware M..B.,.Mujumdar A.M.Ghaskadbi, S., Reproductive toxicity of Piperine in mice., Planta Medica 66(2000) 231- 236.

[70] Chauhan S.K, Kimothi G.P.,. Singh B.P, Agrawal S.., Development of HPLC method to determine piperine in different Piper species, Indian Drugs 35(7), July 1998, 408-411.

developed to estimate piperine in Piper species. This method is simple, rapid, economical, and is based on the identification of piperine by TLC and on the UV absorbance maxima in alcohol at 328 nm[71].

Haridra / Turmeric (*Curcuma longa*)

Haridra (Turmeric) has been studied for effects of curcumin, a yellow pigment of the spice turmeric on the mutagenecity of several environmental mutagens in the Salmonella microsome test with or without Aroctor 1254 induced rat liver homogenate (S-9 mix)[72]. With Salmonella typhimurium strain TA-98 in the presence of S-9 mix curcumin inhibited the mutagenicity of bidi and cigarette smoke condensates, tobacco and masheri extracts benzopyrine and dimethylbenzoanthracene in a dose dependent manner. This indicates that curcumin may alter the metabolic activation and detoxification of mutagens. Curcumin and its derivatives have significant abilities to protect plasmis pBR 322 DNA against single strand breaks induced by singlet oxygen, a reactive oxygen species with potential genotoxic/mutagenic properties. Curcumin was found to be the most effective inhibitor of DNA damage followed by desmethoxycurcumin, bisdesmethoxycurcumin and other derivatives. The observed antioxidant activity was both time and concentration dependent. The protective ability of curcumin was higher than that of well-known biological antioxidants - alpha-tocopherol and beta-carotene. This partly explains the anticarcinogenic and

---

[71] Chauhan S.K, Kimothi G.P., Singh B.P., Agrawal S. A spectrophotometric method to estimate piperine in piper species., Ancient Science of life, Volume 18(1), July 1998, 84-87.

[72] M. Nagabhooshan, A.J.Amonkar, S.V Bhide., In Vitro antimutagenicity of curcumin against environmental mutagens., Fd Chem. Toxic, Vol 25, No 7, 545-547,1987.

antimutagenic properies[73]. High Performance Thin Layer Chromatography method for quantitative analysis of guggul and turmeric has been devised which is precise, specific, reproducible and cost effective[74]. A Spectrophotometric and reverse phase HPLC method to determine curcumin in different samples of *Curcuma longa* has been developed. The linearity in range of 0.1 to 0.8 mcg for HPLC and 2 to 5 mcg for spectophotometric method was observed.

Vidanga (*Embelia ribes*)

Embelin is a plant benzoquinone from berries of *Embelia ribes* with proven antispermatogenic effects. Exposure of male albino rats to embelin forr 15-30 days revealed significant impairment of lipid metabolism. Accumulation of lipid classes in testis, epididymis, and seminal vesicles and prostrate is noted. Administration of embelin results in certain metabolic changes in lipid metabolism in primary and accesory reproductive tissues and serum, which however returns to near normal biochemical make up once the drug regimen, is withdrawn. Although embelin produces functional sterility in the sense that it impairs the production/ maturation of spermatozoa, the withdrawal of treatment results in normalisation of spermatogenic processes and the structural and functional milieu of the reproductive tissues. Thus the compound stands the potential chance of being considered for human welfare by making use of its capability of producing functional sterility

---

[73] Subramaniam M, Sreejayan, Thomas. P.A, Devasagayam, B.B.Singh, Diminution of singlet oxygen induced DNA damage by Curcumin and related antioxidants, Mutation Research 311 (1994) 249.

[74] Sane, R.T. A High Performance Thin Layer Chromatography for the simultaneous quantitative analysis of guggul and turmeric from an Ayurvedic preparation. Indian Drugs 1998; 35(5);286-90.

with reversible mode of action[75]. The biodistribution study of embelin was studied by Gupta *et al.*[76] Administration of embelin in rats by subcutaneous injection or oral route caused significant tissue deposition of drug in testis, epididymis, seminal vesicles, ventral prostrate, liver, kidney, lung, spleen, heart, brain and intestine. Organ weight of the reproductive tissues decreased while it increased weight of non-reproductive tissues. These changes were reversible. Pharmacokinetic studies showed that after subcutaneous administration the fractional turnover rate constant is higher while the biological half-life is shorter thereby indicating faster elimination as compared to oral treatment. Higher concentration was seen in liver and kidney emphasising their role in metabolism and elimination of the drug. The subcutaneous exposure of male albino rats to embelin for 15 to 30 days also reveals significant impairment in carbohydrate metabolism in the primary and secondary reproductive tissues. Alteration of enzyme activities of glycolysis, Kreb's cycle, lipogenesis, NAD and NADP dependent enzymes transaminases and phosphatases are noted in the embelin treated testis, epididymis, seminal vesicles, ventral prostrate as well as spermatozoal suspensions. Marked changes are also noted in levels of glycogen, protein, nucleic acids and certain carbohydrate constituents in these tissues. Reduction in fertility parameters such as pregnancy attainment and litter size obtained is also noted. All these changes are reversed once the drug therapy is withdrawn and the animals are given 15 to 39 days recovery period. Effect of embelin on absorptive and digestive functions of rat intestine was

---

[75] Gupta S., Sanyal S.N.,.Kanwar U, Effects of embelin, an antifertility agent on the lipid metabolism of male albino rats, Fitoterapia, 1989,: Vol LX, No 4, 331-338.

[76] Gupta S., Kanwar U, Biodistribution of embelin, a benzoquinone of male antifertility potential , Fitoterapia, 1991: Vol LXII, No. 5, 419-424.

studied. Oral administration caused significant elevation in uptake of D-glucose, L-alanine, L-leucine and calcium in small intestine segments. Increase in intestinal brush border membrane associated enzymes (sucrase, lactase, maltase etc) and also microsomal glucose 6 phosphatase and cytosolic lactate dehyrogenase and brush border membrane associated total lipids, phospholipids, acholesterol, triacylglycerol, unesterified fatty acids were seen. All these changes returned to control level following drug withdrawal[77]. A TLC method for identification and spectrophotometric method for estimation of embelin has been devised. It is simple, rapid, and economical and can be used for standardization and monitoring of embelin in Embelia ribes[78].

Bramhi (*Bacopa monnieri*)

Bacopa monnieri contains Bacoside A as the active constituent[79]. It is reported to be active in walker carcinoma and the ethanolic extract is toxic to the Sarcoma- 180 cell line[80]. An investigation to confirm the cytotoxic activity was performed in the brine shrimp lethality assay and active constituents were assayed. The ethanol fraction and bacoside A showed potent cytotoxic activity. Bacoside A was responsible for other biological activities also[81]. Anti

---

[77] Gupta S., San yal S.,.Kanwar U, Effects of embelin a male antifertility agent on absorptive and digestive functions of rat intestine, Journal of Ethnopharmacology, 1999: 133, 203-212.

[78] Chauhan S.K.,.Singh B.P and Agrawal S., A spectrophotometric estimation of embelin in Embelia ribes, Ancient Science of Life, Vol XIX, (1 & 2) 46-47.

[79] Bhakuni D. S, Dhar M.L, Mehrothra B, Screening of Indian plants for biological activity, Indian J. of Exp Biol, 1969: 7: 250.

[80] Elangovan V, Govidaswamy .S, Ramamoorthy .N, Balasubramaniam K, In vitro studies of the anticancer activity of Bacopa monnieri, Fitoterapia 1995: 3, 211-215.

[81] D.Souza P, *et al.* Brine shrimp lethality assay of Bacopa monnieri, Phytothe.r Res. 2002: 16, 197-198.

convulsant profile of different extracts of *Bacopa monnieri* in rats was studied using maximum electro shock seizures in rats after administration and pentylene tetrazole (PTZ) test in mice and rats. ED50 dose of Phenytoin (30mg/kg) was used for comparison. Overall Bramhi has faster onset of action and time/dose responses were qualitatively similar to phenytoin. Hence its use as an antiepileptic drug can be supported[82]. Studies on the mast cell stabilising activity of extracts of Bacopa were tested in vitro for mast cell stabilising effects. The methanolic factors exhibited potent activity comparable to disodium cromoglycate, a known mast cell stabiliser. The results indicate its potential use in allergic conditions[83].

Tulsi/Basil (*Ocimum sanctum*)

The essential oil of *Ocimum sanctum* and eugenol tested in vitro showed potent anthelmintic activity in the Caenorhabditis elegans model. The essential oil of Ocimum and eugenol showed potent anthelmintic activity[84]. Oxidative stress is one of the major risk factors for age realted cataract development. Ocimum has natural antioxidants and has been evaluated against galactose induced experimental cataract development in rats. It possesses anti cataract activity[85]. The therapeutic and prophylactic value

---

[82] S.Sudha, S.Kumaresan, A.Amit, S.David, B.V.Venkatraman, Anticonvulsant activity of different extracts of Centenella asiatica and Bacopa monnieri in animals, Journal of Natural remedies Vol 2/1, 33-41, 2002.

[83] Samiullla D.S.,. Prashanth D,. Amit A. Mast cell stabilising activity of Bacopa monnieri, Fitoterapia 2001:72, 284-285.

[84] Asha M.K.,. Prashanth D, Murali B., Padmaja R., Amit A, Anthelmintic activity of essential oil of Ocimum sanctum and eugenol., Fitoterapia, 2001: 72, 669-670.

[85] Srivastava S., Trivedi D., Joshi. S, Halder N, Gupta S.K, Ocimum sanctum- A potential anticataract agent IL 27, Scientific Prog. Abs XXXV Annual Conference of Indian Pharmacological Society, 26-29, Nov 2002.

of *Ocimum sanctum* in treatment of myocardial infarction was evaluated by studying the cardioprotective effeect. Histopathological findings confirmed the cardioprotective effect[86].

Drug Discovery: Intentional Not Coincidental

In the sequence of their appearance, the scientific disciplines involved in drug discovery were: chemistry, pharmacology, physiology, microbiology, biochemistry and molecular biology. It can be shown that new therapeutic classes of drugs like muscle relaxants; diuretics, L-dopa, antibiotics, recombinant proteins, monoclonal antibodies and others were generated on the basis of scientific opportunities rather than therapeutic need. All of these drugs were created within the confines of a chemical paradigm of medicine and drug therapy. We are now witnessing the entry of a new informational paradigm into medicine that is most prominently represented by genomic sciences. This paradigm will bring two important changes to the therapy of diseases. First, molecular biology has matured to such a degree that it can now study complex genomes and their functionality in complex organisms such as humans. Therefore, results from these studies no longer have to be translated into the context of medicine: they are already within this context. Secondly, drug therapy that used to be largely symptomatic, will now aim at targets, which are closer to the causes of diseases than previously. Therapeutic progress, which used to be indirect, conjectural and coincidental, is about to become more directed, definitive and intentional. The future of drug discovery will be more often based on intent rather than coincidence.

---

[86] Sharma Meenu, Kishore Kamal, Gupta Suresh, Joshi Sujata and Arya D. S. Cardioprotective potential of Ocimum sanctum in isoproterenol induced myoccardial infarction in rats 2001, Molecular and Cellular Biochemistry, 225:75-83.

Proper bio-prospecting of medicinal sources will be an important factor[87].

Modern medical science is currently in the phase of a revolution, which is likely to have a dramatic impact on both the theory of medicine and the way it is practiced. The mechanistic model, which served biomedicine well for many years, is gradually collapsing, according to Svoboda (1998). Efforts of dedicated researchers are looking beyond that model's flaws. We now know that networks of chemical communication exist between the nervous and immune systems, and that prayer at a distance can positively affect the conditions of those who are seriously ill, even when the prayer and the patient are not known to one another. Another participant in this exciting climate of change and ferment is Ayurveda, India's ancient medical system. While Ayurveda has already contributed much to modern medicine (reserpine, gugulipid, plastic surgery), its real contributions are yet to be made. While some of these are likely to come in matters of materia medica and technique, the most benefit will likely be derived from Ayurveda's vision of medicine's ability to teach people not just how to avoid disease but how to proactively develop and maintain a healthy state[88]. In practice, Ayurveda is a dynamic phenomenon that offers multifaceted approaches to healing. These diverse healing formats develop to meet the constantly changing needs of the society and of illness patterns. This analysis views illness and health care in terms of the multiple systems of knowledge and action, phenomena and interaction, that characterize them as well

---

[87] Drews J. Intent and coincidence in pharmaceutical discovery. The impact of biotechnology. Arzneimittel Forschung 1995 Aug 45:8 934-9.

[88] Svoboda R. Ayurveda's role in preventing disease.. Indian J Med Sci 1998 Feb 52:2 70-7.

as in terms of the medical treatises and institutions that formalize them. From this perspective, Ayurveda emerges as a plural medical system in itself [89].

Ayurveda: A New Discovery Engine

Combining the strengths of the knowledge base of traditional systems such as Ayurveda with the dramatic power of combinatorial sciences and high throughput screening will help in the generation of structure-activity libraries. Ayurvedic knowledge and experiential database can provide new functional leads to reduce time, money and toxicity— the three main hurdles in the drug development. These records are particularly valuable since effectively these medicines have been tested for thousands years on people[90]. Efforts are underway to establish pharmacoepidemiological evidence-base to Ayurvedic medicines, safety and practice[91]. Development of standardized herbal formulations is underway as an initiative of the Council for Scientific and Industrial Research (CSIR) New Millennium Indian Technology Leadership Initiative (NMITLI). Randomized controlled clinical trials for Rheumatoid and Osteoarthritis, Hepatoprotectives, Hypolipedemic agents, Asthma, Parkinson's disease, and many other disorders have reasonably established clinical efficacy. A review of some exemplary evidence-based researches and approaches has now resulted in wider acceptance of Ayurvedic

---

[89] Nordstrom CR. Exploring pluralism—the many faces of Ayurveda. Soc Sci Med 1988 27:5 479-89.

[90] Patwardhan B and Hooper M. Ayurveda and Future Drug Development. International Journal of Alternative and Complementary Medicine. 1992, 10(12), 9-11.

[91] Vaidya Ashok et al. Ayurvedic pharmacoepidemiology-a new discipline, Journal of Association of Physicians India (JAPI), 2003: 51; 528.

medicines[92,93]. Thus the Ayurvedic knowledge database allows drug researchers to start from a well-tested and safe botanical material. With Ayurveda, the normal drug discovery course of 'Laboratory to Clinics' actually becomes from 'Clinics to Laboratories' — a true Reverse Pharmacology Approach[94]. In this process 'Safety' remains the most important starting point and the efficacy becomes a matter of validation[95]. Globally, there is a positive trend towards holistic health, integrative sciences, systems biology approaches in drug discovery and therapeutics that has remained one of the unique features of Ayurveda[96]. A golden triangle[97] consisting of Ayurveda-Modern medicine - Science will converge to form a real discovery engine that can result in newer, safer, cheaper and effective therapies. It will be in the interest of pharmaceutical companies, researchers and ultimately the global community to respect the traditions and build on their knowledge and experiential wisdom[98].

❏❏❏

---

[92] Chopra A. Lavin P., Patwardhan B, *et al.* Randomized Double Blind Trial of an Ayurvedic Plant Derived Formulation for Treatment of Rheumatoid Arthritis. The Journal of Rheumatology 200; 27:6:1365-1372.

[93] Vaidya A.D.B., Vaidya R.A., Nagaral S.I. Ayurveda and a different level of evidence: From Lord Macaulay to Lord Walton (1835-2001 AD), Journal of Association of Physicians India (JAPI), 2001; 49:534-537.

[94] Ashok Vaidya, Reverse Pharmacology Approach 2002, CSIR-NMITLI Herbal Drug Development Program.

[95] Ayurvedic Medicine: Safety and Validation need. Patwardhan B. National Symposium Ayurvedic. Drug Manufactures Association, New Delhi, 1999.

[96] Nitya Anand, CSIR Golden Diamond Jubilee Symposium on Rasayana Drugs, August 7-8, 2003, CDRI Luchnow.

[97] Mashelkar R.A. Chitrakoot Declaration, National Botanical Research Institute Convention, 2003.

[98] Patwardhan B. *et al.* Herbal remedies and bias against Ayurvedaa. Current Science, 2003: 84(9); 1165.

4 Innovation and Drug Discovery

Contrary to "Law of Finite Biology" though the number of genetic codes will exhaust soon in an exponential way (presumably leading to solutions to every known genetic anomaly related health problem), the number of NCE (New Chemical Entity), their number being finite[99] too, will run out of fuel soon too, despite unraveling of genomic decoding. The bleak scenario in the pharmaceutical field is a testimony to the latter surmise. As many a wise scholar has pointed out, the era of single molecule drug seem to drawing curtains. However, unlike what seems common sense, the era of combinational drug therapies of MM paradigm probably will not foot the bill. Just as very high speed serial computing simulates parallel processing but does not make real time parallel processing, mixtures of prima facie complementary medicinal molecules will perhaps not make combinational recipes. The fundamentals of non-linear dynamical complex systems (NLDCS) paradigm demand so. The odds against success with such efforts are close to odds of success of creating life one bit at a time out of mixing C, H and O molecules in a

[99] Patwardhan Avinash (unpublished work), Refer to WHO CIPIH Report on TM 2005.

jar would be. The number of genes might be finite, but data on their combinations (and their corresponding effects) and more so on their permutations (one has to only imagine the vastness of those possibilities) would, as of now or in near future, cause an information overload and comprehension failure[100] (limitation of human biological brain apparatus) pitting researchers and industry against a futility barrier. However, TM provides a silver lining to these bleak analyses. Analytical comprehension of TM recipes, regimens or techniques might be unachievable by contemporary science, empirical testing of their efficacy and safety being doable and therefore taken care of, TM can provide an outlet to the drug discovery impasse because the same natural forces that shaped multi-gene interaction into complex and dynamical mode have created some of, if not all, TM solutions.

Innovation and Drug Discovery

The age of the blockbuster drug seems over, or at least in its last days. The data from a study done by DiMasi and Paquette of Tufts University, suggest that entry barriers have fallen over time for new drug introductions. The increased competitiveness of the pharmaceutical marketplace was likely fueled by changes over time on both the supply and demand sides. The development histories of entrants to new drug classes suggest that development races better characterize new drug development than does a model of *post hoc* imitation. Thus, the usual distinctions drawn between breakthrough and 'me-too' drugs may not be very meaningful[101]. The pharmaceutical industry has not

---

[100] Patwardhan Avinash (unpublished work)

[101] DiMasi J.A. and Paquette C. The Economics of Follow-on Drug Research and Development Trends in Entry Rates and the Timing of Development Pharmacoeconomics 2004; 22 (2): 1-14.

been as innovative as it claims to be and the regulatory processes are adding more risk and years for the pharmaceutical companies and it is predicated that worst is yet to come[102]. Most of the big pharmaceutical manufacturers spend more on marketing than on research and development. Drug companies actively research for new ways to interact with known receptors and seek out new receptors. But the development road is long, stony, and expensive, as seen in many cases of post approval or marketing withdrawal cases such as a new anticoagulant Ximelagatran of Astra Zeneca[103] or Cox II inhibitor Vioxx of Pfizer[104]. Such failures are really becoming nightmares of pharmaceutical companies who are now looking for innovative approaches to drug discovery. There are common approaches to drug discovery including Chemical Biology Approach, Serendipity and Synthetic, Combinatorial, Genomics Approaches. However, the innovative approaches based on TM that are evolving to reduce major bottleneck and to reduce cost and development time, include Ethnopharmacology Approach, Reverse Pharmacology Approach, Systems Biology Approach and Personalized Approach[105,106].

---

[102] The Economist, Nov 25th 2004,The pharmaceuticals industry From bad to awful.

[103] Briefing Information, US Food and Drug Administration, Cardiovascular and Renal Drugs Advisory Committee, September 10, 2004.

[104] Kweder Sandra, Office of New Drugs, Center for Drug Evaluation and Research, U.S. Food and Drug Administration, statement before - Committee on Finance United States Senate, regarding worldwide withdrawal by Merck & Co., Inc. of Vioxx. November 18, 2004.

[105] Patwardhan B. Symposium on TM, Annual Meeting of Indian Academy of Sciences, Varanasi India, 2004.

[106] CSIR-NMITLI Herbal Drug Development Program, Government of India, 2001-2005.

The traditional route to drug discovery, the old pharmacology of testing analogues of active drugs or the slightly newer pharmacology of mass screenings in chemical libraries, is not yet over, but neither has rational drug come up with a blockbuster, although it may do one day. The challenge is set for drug companies to become truly innovative. A good start would be to forget the me-too market and to go and find those receptors, old and new, and the genuinely new compounds to interact with them[107]. There are clear trends that show the mainstream pharmaceutical research is moving away from single molecule or single target approach in favor of combinations and multiple target approaches[108].

Thus, in the current scenario, TM knowledge database has considerable potential that remains under explored and poorly understood. Developing countries could exploit traditional medicine to kick-start biotech, only if their products measure up to the demands of Western regulators. For example, the traditional Chinese medicine - Kanglaite Injection is ready to enter Phase II clinical trials in the United States for the treatment of several cancers, including breast and prostate cancer[109]. A standardized herbal formulation for treatment of psoriasis developed by Lupin Ltd of India presents a good case where the company has filed several Patents and IND application in India and USA. In short, for several reasons, the modern drug discovery processes have started revisiting TM to reduce the typical innovation

---

[107] Editorial, The Lancet, 2004, 364; 1100.

[108] Camille Wermuth, Multitargeted drugs: The end of the one-target-one disease philosophy? Drug Discovery Today 19, October 2004.

[109] Basu P. Trading on traditional medicines, Nature Biotechnology 2004, 22, 263 – 265.

deficit faced today that would help reaching to the top in Sciences especially for developing counties like India[110].

TM knowledge and experiential database can provide new functional leads to reduce time, money and toxicity - the three main hurdles in the drug development. These records are particularly valuable since effectively these medicines have been tested for thousands years on people[111]. Efforts are underway to establish pharmacoepidemiological evidence-base to TM, safety and practice[112]. Combining the strengths of the knowledge base of traditional systems with the dramatic power of combinatorial sciences and high throughput screening will help in the generation of structure-activity libraries. Development of standardized herbal formulations is underway as an initiative of the Council for Scientific and Industrial Research (CSIR) is playing an important role through public-private profiting partnerships in R&D in a very professional manner and has received due appreciation from the corporate, scientific and governmental sectors[113] and its program known as New Millennium Indian Technology Leadership Initiative (NMITLI)[114] and a CORE Network Projects[115] involving 21 leading national laboratories, Universities and hospitals has claimed several leads in short time. Most of these efforts innovate on existing knowledgebase complemented with

---

[110] Mashelkar R.A., 2005. Global Voices of Science: India's R&D: Reaching for the Top. Science, 307 (5714), 1415-1417.

[111] Patwardhan B and Hooper M. Ayurvedaa and Future Drug Development. International Journal of Alternative and Complementary Medicine. 1992, 10(12), 9-11.

[112] Vaidya Ashok et al. Ayurvedic pharmacoepidemiology-a new discipline, Journal of Association of Physicians India (JAPI), 2003: 51; 528.

[113] Jolly VK. Profiting from R&D, in World Class India Ed Ghosal S *et. al.*, Penguin Books India, 2001.

[114] Rao Yogeshwar, Technology Network and Business Development Division, CSIR, New Delhi.

[115] Agarwal O.P. , CORE Network Projects, CSIR, New Delhi.

cutting edge technologies for drug discovery and developments mainly based on TM. Randomized controlled clinical trials for Rheumatoid and Osteoarthritis, Hepatoprotectives, Diabetes, Hypolipedemic agents, Asthma, Parkinson's disease, and many other disorders have reasonably established clinical efficacy. Many CSIR laboratories are active in research and development efforts and innovations related to TM. The Regional Research Laboratory (RRL) Jammu, National Chemical Laboratory (NCL), Pune, Central Botanical Research Institute (NBRI) and Central Institute of Medicinal and Aromatic Plants (CIMAP) Lucknow, Institute of Himalian Bioprospecting Technology, Palampur, Indian Institute of Chemical Biology Kolkata, Indian Institute of Chemical Technology, Hyderabad are just few examples. There is growing Industry-Academia partnerships in this field, which is a good indication. For instance, in the NMITLI program of Government of India: number of industry partners such as Nicholas Piramal, Lupin, Zandu, Dabur, Dhootpapeshwar, Natural Remedies, are part of the project. A review of some exemplary evidence-based researches and approaches has now resulted in wider acceptance of Ayurvedic medicines[116,117,118]. Research laboratories such as RRL, NBRI and CIMAP have done some innovations through R&D contributions in traditional medicines[119]. One of the

---

[116] Chopra A. Lavin P., Patwardhan B, *et al.* Randomized Double Blind Trial of an Ayurvedic Plant Derived Formulation for Treatment of Rheumatoid Arthritis. The Journal of Rheumatology 200; 27:6:1365-1372.

[117] Vaidya A.D.B., Vaidya R.A., Nagaral S.I. Ayurveda and a different level of evidence: From Lord Macaulay to Lord Walton (1835-2001 AD), Journal of Association of Physicians India (JAPI), 2001; 49:534-537.

[118] Patwardhan B and Gautam M, 2005. Botanical Immunodrugs: Scope and Opportunities. Drug Discovery Today 10 (7/24), 495-502.

[119] Research projects of CIMAP at www.csir.res.in.

bioenhancers developed by RRL is Piperine, which has been studied in detail with anti-TB drugs[120]. The development of artemisinin and its derivatives, development of superior varieties like Jeevan Raksha and CIM-Arogya producing significantly higher yields of artemisnin, with complete package of agrotechnology. CIMAP has worked on bio-enhancers that could reduce the dosage of antibiotics and subsequently the toxicity. A new antibiotic Oenostacin from the roots of the plant *Oenothera biennis* has been found effective. A new synergistic combination comprising of essential oil of medicinal plant *Foenicum vulgare* and other plants has been found to be effective as an insecticide against mosquito larvae and has toxic action against larval stages of malarial vector, *Anopheles stephensi*.

Thus the TM knowledge database allows drug researchers to start from a well-tested and safe botanical material. With Ayurveda, the normal drug discovery course of 'Laboratory to Clinics' actually becomes from 'Clinics to Laboratories'— a true Reverse Pharmacology Approach[121]. A brief description of Reverse Pharmacology approach and how it could save time, cost and toxicity the tree main bottlenecks in drug discovery is given later in this report as a case study. In this process 'Safety' remains the most important starting point and the efficacy becomes a matter of validation[122] Globally, there is a positive trend towards holistic health, integrative sciences, systems biology approaches in drug discovery and therapeutics that has

---

[120] A Process For The Preparation Of Pharmaceutical Composition With Enhanced Activity For The Treatmet Of Tuberculosis And Leprosy: Patents- In 172689 ; Us 0650728; Ep 93308653.

[121] Ashok Vaidya, Reverse Pharmacology Approach 2002, CSIR-NMITLI Herbal Drug Development Program.

[122] Ayurvedic Medicine: Safety and Validation need. Patwardhan B. National Symposium Ayurvedic. Drug Manufactures Association, New Delhi, 1999.

remained one of the unique features of Ayurveda[123]. A golden triangle[124] consisting of Ayurveda-Modern medicine - Science will converge to form a real discovery engine that can result in newer, safer, cheaper and effective therapies. It will be in the interest of pharmaceutical companies, researchers and ultimately the global community to respect the traditions and build on their knowledge and experiential wisdom[125]. Most important fact is Traditions do not mean just drugs or medicine, they are based on philosophical and experiencial principles and practices. An ambitious innovative project to study some of the important basic principles and practices of Ayurveda using most advanced tools of science has been conceived under the name 'Science Initiatives in Ayurveda'. This program is being supported by the Principal Scientific Advisor's Office, Government of India and involves premeum national institutes such as IITs, IISc, TIFR and Universities including Pune and Banaras[126].

The R&D thrust, in the pharmaceutical sector is focused on development of new drugs, innovative/ indigenous processes for known drugs and development of plant based drugs through investigation of leads from the traditional systems of medicine. This is happening at the drawback of a great innovation deficit that pharmaceutical industry is currently facing. In addition, many nutraceuticals are being consumed in unregulated markets for perceived benefits in health care and improvement of quality of life. Natural pharmaceuticals,

---

[123] Nitya Anand, CSIR Golden Diamond Jubilee Symposium on Rasayana Drugs, August 7-8, 2003, CDRI Luchnow.

[124] Mashelkar R.A. Chitrakoot Declaration, National Botanical Research Institute Convention, 2003.

[125] Patwardhan B. *et al.* Ayurvedaa and Natural Product Drug Discovery. Current Science, 2004: 86(6); 789-799.

[126] Valiathan MS, Science Initiatives in Ayurveda, PSA and DST, Government of India, 2006.

nutraceuticals and cosmeceuticals are of great importance as a reservoir of chemical diversity aimed at new drug discovery and are explored for antimicrobial, cardiovascular, immunosuppressive, and anticancer drugs. Around 80% of all such products are of plant origin; their sales exceeded $ 65 billion in 2003. Examples of plant products and derivatives used by the pharmaceutical industry include Paclitaxel, Vincristine, Vinblastine, Artemisinin, Camptothecin, Podophyllotoxin, etc. The nutraceutical marketplace in Europe is estimated to be $ 9 billion, while the US marketplace, estimated to be $10-12 billion in 2003, is expanding at a compounded rate of more than 20% per year. The rapid growth of nutraceuticals in the US led to the Dietary Supplement Health and Education Act (DSHEA) in 1994. Globally, there have been efforts to monitor quality and regulate the growing business of herbal drugs and traditional medicine[127].

Thirty percent of the worldwide sales of drugs are based on natural products. Though recombinant proteins and peptides account for increasing sales rates, the superiority of low-molecular mass compounds in human diseases therapy remains undisputed mainly due to more favorable compliance and bioavailability properties. Approaches to improve and accelerate the joint drug discovery and development process are expected to take place mainly from innovation in drug target elucidation and lead structure discovery. Therefore, need for new concepts to generate large compounds collection with improved structural diversity has been correctly emphasized[128]. There are number of problems connected

---

[127] Prakash P. 2nd Nutraceutical Summit, CFTRI Conference, February 3-5, 2005, New Delhi.

[128] Grabley S; Thiericke R, Bioactive agents from natural sources: trends in discovery and application. Adv Biochem Eng Biotechnol 1999;64:101-54.

with the search for new prototype drugs of biological origin. Investigations of plants used in traditional and modern medicine in China serve as a source of inspiration and as models for the synthesis of new drugs with better therapeutic, chemical or physical properties than the original compounds[129]. The World Health Organization also has recognized the importance of traditional medicine and has been active in creating strategies, guidelines and standards for botanical medicines[130].

Commercially, these plant-derived medicines are worth about $14 billion a year in the United States and $40 billion worldwide. Americans paid an estimated $21.2 billion for services provided by alternative medicine practitioners[131]. A 1997 survey estimated that over 12% of adults had used herbal medicine during 1996 as compared with 2.5% in 1990 resulting a business of $5.1 billion[132]. Lilly Research Laboratories markets several million dollars worth of Vincristine and Vinblastine – the periwinkle derivatives used to treat childhood leukemia and Hodgkin's disease. The U.S. National Cancer Institute regularly earmarks large appropriations to screen 50,000 natural substances for activity against cancer cell lines and the AIDS virus. China, Germany, India, and Japan, among others, are also screening wild species for new drugs.

---

[129] Baerheim SA and; Scheffer JJ. Natural products in therapy. Prospects, goals and means in modern research., Pharm Weekl [Sci] 1982 Aug 20;4(4): 93-103.

[130] W.H.O. Traditional Medicine Strategy 2002-2005, W.H.O. Geneva, 2002.

[131] Eisenberg D.M. *et. al,* Trends in alternative medicine use in US, The Journal of the American Medical Association, 1998 November 11.

[132] De Smet, Herbal Remedies, The New England Journal of Medicine, 2002: 347: 2046-2056.

Proven agro-industrial technologies need to be applied to the cultivation and processing of medicinal plants and the manufacture of herbal medicines[133]. The mass screening of plants in the search for new drugs is vastly expensive and inefficient. It would be cheaper and perhaps more productive to re-examine plant remedies described in ancient and mediaeval texts[134]. Many higher plants produce economically important organic compounds such as oils, resins, tannins, natural rubber, gums, waxes, dyes, flavors, fragrances, pharmaceuticals, and pesticides. Advances in biotechnology, particularly methods for culturing plant cells and tissues, should provide new means for the commercial processing of even rare plants and the chemicals they produce. These new technologies will extend and enhance the usefulness of plants as renewable resources of valuable chemicals. In the future, biologically active plant-derived chemicals can be expected to play an increasingly significant role in the commercial development of new products for regulating plant growth and for insect and weed control[135].

In the natural product drug discovery it is important to follow systems-theory and systems biology applications

---

[133] Akerele O. Nature's medicinal bounty: don't throw it away. W.H.O. Geneva, Switzerland. World Health Forum 1993; 14(4): 390-5.

[134] Holland BK. Prospecting for drugs in ancient texts. Nature 1994 Jun 30; 369 (6483), Comment in Nature 1994 Sep 1; 371 (6492): 9, Comment in: Nature 1994 Nov 10; 372 (6502): 124; Comment in: Nature 1995 Aug 17; 376 (6541): 546; Cox PA. The ethnobotanical approach to drug discovery. Scientific American 1994 Jun; 270(6): 82.

[135] Balandrin MF; Klocke JA; Wurtele ES; Bollinger WH. Natural plant chemicals: sources of industrial and medicinal materials. Science 1985 Jun 7; 228(4704): 1154-60]; Bonati A,. Medicinal plants and industry.

J. Ethnopharmacol 1980 Jun; 2(2): 167-71; Wijesekera RO. Is there an industrial future for phytopharmaceutical drugs? An outline of UNIDO programs in the sector. Chemical Industries Branch, United Nations Industrial Development Organization. J Ethnopharmacol 1991 Apr; 32(1-3): 217-24.

to facilitate the process[136]. Routine random efforts are not likely to increase the desired success rate of discovery while experience indicates that a modified collection policy offered better chances for the discovery and development of agents for treatment of AIDS and cancer[137]. Numerous drugs have entered the international pharmacopoeia via of ethnobotany and traditional medicine[138]. There are many similarities in traditional systems of medicine as well as ethnomedicines being connected to each other as 'great traditions and little traditions'. All botanical drugs will have to fulfill the international requirements on quality, safety and efficacy[139].

Efficacy and Evidence

Efficacy of TM is one of the most debated issues. There are philosophical, cultural, technical, methodological and practical aspects involved in efficacy evaluation. Reports of investigations of their clinical efficacy or otherwise have been published in prestigious international scientific journals. For instance, the efficacy of acupuncture in relieving pain and nausea has been well demonstrated and

---

[136] Leroy Hood, Principles, Practice and Future of Systems Biology, Drug Discovery Today 2003: 8(10); 436-438.

[137] Cragg GM; Boyd MR; Cardellina JH 2nd; Newman DJ; Snader KM; McCloud. Ethnobotany and drug discovery: the experience of the US National Cancer Institute Developmental Therapeutics Program, National Cancer Institute, Bethesda, Ciba Foundation Symposium 1994;185:178-90; 190-96. Kitagawa I, Elucidation of scientific basis for traditional medicines and exploitation of new naturally occurring drugs, Yakugaku Zasshi 1992 Jan 112:1 1-41.

[138] De Smet PA, The role of plant-derived drugs and herbal medicines in healthcare. Drugs 1997 Dec; 54(6): 801-40; King SR; Tempesta MS. From shaman to human clinical trials: the role of industry in ethnobotany, conservation and community reciprocity. Ciba Found Symp 1994; 185:197-206; discussion 206-13.

[139] Vogel HG. Similarities between various systems of traditional medicine: Considerations for the future of ethnopharmacology, J. Ethnopharmacol 1991 Dec 35:2 179-90.

is now acknowledged worldwide. For herbal medicines, some of the best-known evidence for efficacy of an herbal product includes *Artemisia annua* for the treatment of malaria, St John's wort for the management of mild to moderate depression. Patients usually experience fewer side effects than when treated with antidepressants, such as amitriptyline. Such findings have inspired research worldwide to establish the efficacy of other extensively used TM. Many plant extracts have a variety of pharmacological effects, including anti-inflammatory, vasodilatory, antimicrobial, anticonvulsant, sedative and antipyretic effects. However, very few randomized-controlled studies have been carried out to investigate the practice and treatment delivery of herbal practitioners in their everyday work. Regarding non-medication therapies, the 1999 *British Medical Journal* series on CAM commented that randomized controlled trials have provided good evidence that both hypnosis and relaxation techniques can reduce anxiety, and prevent panic disorders and insomnia. Randomized trials have also shown hypnosis to be of value in treating asthma and irritable bowel syndrome, yoga to be of benefit in asthma, and tai ji in helping elderly people to reduce their fear of falls. Besides these limitations, there has been enormous research that has been and is underway in many institutions globally. Many of the findings do substantiate the traditional claims. Many of such studies have been published in peer-reviewed journals with good impact factors. This report has tried to take some representative examples of such evidence for efficacy of TM. Due to limited space, many important findings, observations, reports, patents and such other documentation may be missing, however, that does not adversely reflect on their importance. For instance, details of most studied medicinal plant like Ginseng are not covered here. Similarly, many patents, scientific reports and clinical trials of many important diseases such as AIDS are missing here. This will remain one of the limitation of this study and is mainly due to space constrain. Following are few representative examples of recent studies related to evidence of efficacy.

Ginkgo biloba

In a randomized, double blind, placebo controlled comparison of *Ginkgo biloba* and acetazolamide for prevention of acute mountain sickness among Himalayan trekkers for the prevention of high altitude illness could not establish efficacy significantly different from placebo for any outcome; however participants in the acetazolamide group showed significant levels of protection. When compared with placebo, ginkgo was not effective at preventing acute mountain sickness while, Acetazolamide afforded robust protection against symptoms of acute mountain sickness[140]. A case of persistent postoperative bleeding following total hip arthroplasty was reported to be due to its anticoagulant that inhibits platelet-activating factor, which is contraindicated with aspirin[141]. In a recent case study, side effects such as bilateral haematoma of chronic treatment with *Ginkgo biloba* following rhytidoplasty and blepharoplasty are reported[142].

Uncaria tomentosa

Also known as cat's claw, is from the highlands of the Peruvian Amazon, and has been used by natives for

---

[140] Jeffrey H *et. al.*, BMJ, doi:10.1136/bmj.38043.501690.7C (published 11 March 2004).

[141] Bebbington A. Persistent bleeding after total hip arthroplasty caused by herbal self-medication Journal of Arthroplasty 2005; 20(1) 125-126.

[142] Destro M. W. B. Bilateral haematoma after rhytidoplasty and blepharoplasty following chronic use of Ginkgo biloba British Journal of Plastic Surgery 2005; 58 (1); 100-101.

hundreds of years to treat immunologic and digestive disorders. It was found that two chemo types of Uncaria tomentosa with different alkaloid patterns occur in nature. Aqueous extracts and mixtures of oxindole alkaloids have shown positive influence on IL-1, IL-6 and IFN gamma production suggesting immunoregulatory activity. In one of clinical studies, extract exhibited immune adjuvant activity with pneumococcal vaccine resulting in enhanced lymphocyte/neutrophil ratio and persistent antibody titer responses towards different pneumococcal serotypes[143]. In vitro, in vivo and gene expression studies on extracts of this plant indicated that anti-inflammatory activity is mediated through negation of NF-kappa activation and TNF alpha synthesis suppression[144]. Randomized clinical studies on a purified extract, rich in pentacyclic alkaloids, demonstrated safer and moderate benefit in patients with active RA compared with those taking sulfasalazine[145].

Echinacea Spp.

The *Echinacea* plant is a member of the *Compositae* family; the three species of medicinal interest include *Echinacea angustifolia, Echinacea purpurea,* and *Echinacea pallida.* Most uses of *E. purpurea* are based on its reported immunological properties. There are four types of constituents purported to be pharmacologically active molecules: phenolic caffeic acid derivatives, alkylamides/

---

[143] Winkler, C. *et. al.*, (2004) In vitro effects of two extracts and two pure alkaloid preparations of Uncaria tomentosa on peripheral blood mononuclear cells. Planta Med. 70, 205-10.

[144] Sandoval, M. *et. al.*, (2000) Cat's claw inhibits TNF alpha production and scavenges free radicals: role in cytoprotection. Free Radic Biol Med. 29, 71-8.

[145] Mur, E. *et. al.*, (2002) Randomized double blind trial of an extract from the pentacyclic alkaloid-chemotype of Uncaria tomentosa for the treatment of rheumatoid arthritis. J Rheumatol. 29, 678-81.

isobutylamides, polysaccharides and glycoproteins. Several randomized trials have reported health benefits of *Echinacea* extracts in upper respiratory tract infections[146].

Withania somnifera

Withania somnifera (WS), known as *ashwagandha*, Indian ginseng, and winter cherry is also classified as Rasayana in Ayurveda. The major biochemical constituents of WS root are steroidal alkaloids and steroidal lactones known as withanolides. Several preclinical studies have examined cytoprotective, immunomodulatory and immunoadjuvant potential of WS[147]. WS exhibited modulatory effects on cytotoxic lymphocytes production leading to reduce tumor growth. WS treatment in normal and tumor bearing mice resulted positive influence on natural killer cells activity resulting in enhanced cell killing[148,149]. In a comparative pharmacological investigation of WS and Ginseng, WS treated group showed better anabolic and antistress activity than Ginseng with additional anti-inflammatory activity. Clinical studies on WS have shown moderate analgesic, anti-inflammatory and disease modifying activity in arthritis patients[150].

---

[146] Henneicke-von, Z. H. *et. al.*, (1999) Efficacy and safety of a fixed combination phytomedicine in the treatment of the common cold (acute viral respiratory tract infection): results of a randomised, double blind, placebo controlled, multicentric study. Curr Med Res Opin. 15, 214-227.

[147] Gautam, M. *et. al.*, (2004) Immune response modulation to DPT vaccine by aqueous extract of Withania somnifera in experimental system. Int Immunopharmacol. 4, 841-849.

[148] Diwanay, S. *et. al.*, (2004) Immunoprotection by botanical drugs in cancer chemotherapy. J Ethnopharmacol. 90, 49-55.

[149] Jayaprakasam, B *et. al.*, (2003) Growth inhibition of human tumor cell lines by withanolides from Withania somnifera leaves. Life Sci 74,125-32.

[150] Chopra A, *et. al.*, (2000) Randomized double blind trial of an Ayurvedic plant derived formulation for treatment of rheumatoid arthritis. J. Rheum. 27, 365-72.

Traditional Spices

A typical oriental traditional diet includes a variety of spices such as black pepper, long pepper, ginger and turmeric. A considerably research has supported antioxidant, immunomodulatory and bioavailablity enhancer activity of such spices[151]. For instance, turmeric, which is dietary staple of India, has been used as a home remedy for number of ailments including wound healing. Alzheimer's disease rates are reportedly among the world's lowest in India where turmeric is routinely consumed. Yang and coworkers from University of California Medical School have recently published scientific evidence in support of this. They reported curcumin to block and break up brain plaques that cause the Alzheimer's disease. This spice has also been found to correct the cystic fibrosis defect in mice, prevent the onset of alcoholic liver disease and may slow down the blood cancer multiple myeloma as well as multiple sclerosis[152]. Anti-invasive gene expression studies and modulation of human multi-drug resistance MDR 1 gene by active ingredient of turmeric (curminoids) has been reported[153,154]. Active ingredients of ginger (gingerols) have been reported as a new class of vanilloid receptor agonists[155,156]. In short, there is good level of experimental

---

[151] Regional Research Laboratory Jammu, India Publications and Patents.

[152] Yang F. *et. al.,* 2005. Curcumin inhibits formation of A-beta oligomers and fibrils and binds plaques and reduces amyloid in vivo. J. Biol. Chem, 10.1074.

[153] Chen H.W. Anti-invasive gene expression profile of curcumin in lung adenocarcinoma based on a high throughput microarray analysis. Mol Pharmacol. 2004; 65(1): 99-110.

[154] Limtrakul P, Modulation of human multidrug-resistance MDR-1 gene by natural curcuminoids. BMC Cancer. 2004 Apr 17; 4(1): 13.

[155] Dedov VN. Gingerols: a novel class of vanilloid receptor (VR1) agonists. Br J Pharmacol. 2002 Nov; 137(6): 793-8.

[156] Ohizumi et al. Stimulation of sarcoplasmic reticulum Ca (2+)-ATPase by gingerol analogues. Biol Pharm Bull. 1996 Oct; 19(10): 1377-9.

evidence to support various claims and advantages of various spices used in traditional diet and TM.

Malaria

Traditional medicines have been used to treat malaria for thousands of years and are the source of the two main groups (artemisinin and quinine derivatives) of modern antimalarial drugs. With the problems of increasing levels of drug resistance coupled with affordability and access to effective antimalarial drugs, traditional medicines are considered as an important and sustainable source of treatment. The Research Initiative on Traditional Antimalarial Methods (RITAM) has conducted systematic literature reviews and prepared guidelines aiming to standardize and improve the quality of ethnobotanical, pharmacological, and clinical studies on herbal antimalarials including plant based methods of insect repellence and vector control[157].

Osteoarthritis

This degenerative disease has high prevalence both in developing and developed countries. Current therapies are mostly symptomatic targeted towards pain management. Glucosamine and Chondrantin sulphate have been in use as nutritional supplements, however, there are mixed efficacy outcomes. NIH has funded one of the large multicentric clinical studies and the current reported data does not support in favor[158]. A moderate efficacy of Indian Ayurvedic formulation has been established in a

[157] Willcox Merlin L, Bodeker Gerard, Traditional herbal medicines for malaria, BMJ 2004; 329:1156–9

[158] Cibere J, Randomized, double-blind, placebo-controlled glucosamine discontinuation trial in knee osteoarthritis. Arthritis Rheum. 2004 Oct 15;51(5):738-45.

randomized controlled clinical trial[159]. Acupuncture as a complementary therapy to the pharmacological treatment of osteoarthritis of the knee has also been studied in a randomised controlled trial[160]. Results of this study on 88 patients demonstrated that Acupuncture plus diclofenac is more effective than placebo acupuncture plus diclofenac for the symptomatic treatment of osteoarthritis of the knee.

Eczema

Efficacy and tolerability of borage oil in adults and children with atopic eczema was studied in randomised, double blind, placebo controlled, parallel group trial. No significant differences occurred between treatment groups in the other assessments. Subset analysis of adults and children did not indicate any difference in response. Although, the treatments were well tolerated, linolenic acid was not found beneficial in atopic dermatitis[161].

Obesity

Over the 12-week trial, subjects on the active treatment experienced significantly greater weight loss than subjects on placebo, without an increase in blood pressure, pulse, or the rate of adverse events. These benefits were achieved in the absence of any lifestyle treatment to change dietary or exercise behavior and with lower doses of ephedrine alkaloids and caffeine than those commonly utilized[162].

Such mixed responses make a case for TM more difficult to sustain on the evidence-based approaches. There

---

[159] Chopra *et. al.*, Journal of Rheumatology 2000; J Clin Rheumatology 2004

[160] José María León *et. al.*, BMJ 2004;329;1216.

[161] Takwale A *et. al.*, BMJ 2003;327;1385-89.

[162] Coffey C S *et. al.*, A randomized double-blind placebo-controlled clinical trial of a product containing ephedrine, caffeine, and other ingredients from herbal sources for treatment of overweight and obesity in the absence of lifestyle treatment International Journal of Obesity (2004) 28, 1411-1419.

are divided opinions on usefulness of RCTs in evaluating efficacy of TM. The placebo response remains a vital issue[163]. Particularly in case of psychosomatic conditions some of the clinical trials have reported considerable placebo response to the extent of 40% or even more. This makes the independent assessment of efficacy more difficult. There are very few studies where TM has won over placebo. On the other hand, it is argued that TM needs entirely different methodology and the randomized, placebo controlled model is not suitable or apt to evaluate true effects of TM. The typical pyramid of evidence base where there is due consideration to traditional observational and actual use is arguably important. Many a times traditional practitioners and more so the healers, do not maintain clinical records. What weight one should give to traditional or observational experiences and how to bring in consistency and objectivity in clinical studies on TM still remains to be attended satisfactorily. The pharmacoepidemiological studies become important in such situations[164].

❑❑❑

[163] The Science of Placebo, BMJ Publication 2003.

[164] Vaidya R. *et al.* Ayurvedic Pharmacoepidemiology, J. Asso. Physicians India 2003

5 Bioprospecting and IPR

Ethnopharmacology and Traditional medines use natural resources as medicines. They have developed the knowledge of this through the generations of traditions and experiences. Therefore the protection of this knowledge and protection of natural resources both remain critical. Bioprospecting involves sustainable, ethical and legal processes to access natural resources and use them judicially so that the business needs do not pose any threat to nature and to people.

One important consideration is assuring the preservation of traditional knowledge, particularly oral knowledge, within communities, for the potential benefit of others. Developing mechanisms to document traditional knowledge, such as national inventories, can be beneficial in identifying cases where conservation or cultivation is needed, based on an understanding of existing natural resources used for medicinal purposes. Decisions about access and ownership of information can also be made (including those relating to intellectual property rights, where appropriate) once methods have been found to collect and preserve traditional knowledge. On the other hand, the livelihood of traditional healers may depend on maintaining the secrecy of their healing methods - one argument for consulting with traditional healers as part of the process of planning and executing the collection, storage and testing of traditional medicines.

Extending some form of intellectual property protection to traditional knowledge, of which traditional medical knowledge is a significant part, is being actively debated in WIPO and other international forums. Existing intellectual property regimes can offer protection for purified compounds (produced by scientists and companies) isolated from a natural medicine. But traditional medicines, whose method of action may not be well understood, and which often consist of mixtures of different active substances, may not meet criteria for patentability. The principal impetus for international debate is a desire to compensate the holders of traditional knowledge appropriately for the use of their knowledge by others, or to prevent so-called "biopiracy" where knowledge or genetic materials are used without the consent of the holder. China and Kenya are examples of countries that have modified their laws in an effort to accommodate traditional medicine. It is not intended that the Commission should enter into this debate, except in so far as aspects of it may be relevant to its terms of reference, in particular stimulating innovation in traditional medicine with the purpose of expanding access to affordable medicines.

In a utopia, IPR would belong to entire humanity. But we are far from being there. Until globalization, that began in a real sense after World War II and gathered unprecedented tempo in last three or so decades, IPR landscape was fairly stable if not utterly calm. Like any other industry, pharmaceutical goes by the rule that industry must make profit and expand it, or, at its worst maintain it in a *status quo*. Market and regulatory incentives are two slopes towards which production and its precursors gravitate. Demand backed by affordability (at least true until recently) in the western world drove the pharmaceutical industry to be highly innovative and the IPR protection of market economy in the form of patent monopolies fueled the progress.

Scholars like Dean Baker[165] and Aidan Hollis[166] have argued that monopolies cause prices of drugs to go 400% to at times 1000% above the fair market prices. Excessive money expenditure on marketing, disproportionate increase in production of follow on me-too drugs (what does this phrase mean?), decrease in production of non-patentable drugs, and secretiveness about research sharing and are all explanations for how dysfunction in pharmaceutical markets can inhibit drug research and development. On the other hand, one may argue in concurrence with Kevin Hasset's[167] eloquent article that to let market forces determine drug prices will make them have a better pay off at the bottom line because price control lowers the revenue, which in turn lowers R & D investment and reduces the rate at which new compounds are discovered. To a reader, while both sides and their arguments seem equally convincing, she/he cannot fail to notice that 1. The frame of reference for both schools is western developed countries and 2. Both schools make exclusive economic argument, discounting the purely scientific or technical-technological odds.

One of the most unsettling facts that modern pharmaceutical industry faces is that lately its pipeline of new drug discovery seems to have almost dried up. It seems that the R & D has reached a point of saturation. On the other hand disease prevalence, general economy, and IPR regulations in the developing countries have deviated so

---

165 Financial drug research: What area the issues? CEPR September 2004.

166 Aidan Hollis October 2004.

167 Hassett K. Two Trillion in Ten Years, Wall Street Journal, July 27, 2004.

much from their counter parts in the developed world that they have set up a vicious no win situation for the pharmaceutical industry. To make the matters worse, within developed countries themselves, the segment of Price Controlling Countries[168] is growing larger by the day making the bottleneck tighter still.

Learning from nature its device of selectively permeable membranes/gates/channels[169], perhaps we need to create a new paradigm for IPR that is holistic in orientation where the entire humanity sacrifices some so that the entire humanity survives, thrives and progresses. The slack given to developing countries, for dealing with diseases rampant in their regions, while investing in R & D in developed world to treat those conditions and then passing the fruits to the needy with minimal IPR barriers will only help the entire humanity. On the more upbeat side TMs need to be given the same IPR latitude that was given to modern pharmaceuticals once (that enabled them to become what they have come to be). TMs, as the countries where they originate, are like a growing baby, just as once MM was.

Intellectual Property

According to World Intellectual Property Organization (WIPO), traditional knowledge systems are frameworks for continuing creativity and innovation in most fields of technology, ranging from traditional medicinal plants and agricultural practices, to music[170,171]. Traditional medical

[168] Patented Medicine Prices Review Board, Canada <http://www.pmprb-cepmb.gc.ca/english/view.asp?x=132&mid=57>.

[169] Cellular biology.

[170] WIPO Report on Fact Finding Missions on Intellectual Property Needs and Expectations of Traditional Knowledge Holders. Geneva, April 2001.

[171] Tambutoh D.J. *et. al.,* Traditional medicine and intellectual property rights – a move towards protection in developing countries? WIPO Specialization Course on Intellectual Property, Turin, September 3 – November 29, 2001.

knowledge remains poorly documented. It is mostly transmitted from one generation to the other and is part of the cultural heritage in most developing countries. It has been defined by the WHO Traditional Medicine Program as the sum total of the knowledge, skills and practices based on theories, beliefs, and experiences indigenous to different cultures, whether explicable or not, used in the maintenance of health, as well as in the prevention, diagnosis, improvement or treatment of physical and mental illness. The terms complementary/alternative/non-conventional medicine are used interchangeably with traditional medicine in some countries[172]. The importance of Traditional Medicine in developing countries cannot be over-emphasized as indigenous people cannot survive or exercise their fundamental human rights as distinct nations, societies and people without the ability to conserve, revive, develop and teach the wisdom they have inherited from their ancestors[173]. The Principle 22 of the Rio Declaration states that 'indigenous people and their communities have a vital role in environmental management and development because of their knowledge and traditional practices'.

The significance of this concern becomes evident in connection with the discussion of article 8(j) of the Convention on Biological Diversity 1992, where it is implied that medicinal plants, blood samples from indigenous people and research conducted by foreigners into indigenous ways of life, supported by indigenous possessors of traditional knowledge, have led to patentable discoveries of benefit solely to those foreign researchers, with no economic return to indigenous people themselves[174]. The

[172] WIPO Intellectual Property Handbook: Policy, Law, and Use (2001), Geneva, p. 58, § 2.269.

[173] Protection of the Heritage of Indigenous People, United Nation, New York & Geneva (1997).

[174] UNESCO/WIPO Regional Consultations on the Protection of Traditional and Popular Culture (Folklore), UNESCO Activities, June 1999, p. 38-39.

traditional medical knowledge of indigenous peoples throughout the world has played an important role in identifying biological resources worthy of commercial exploitation[175]. Knowledge about the way in which local people have used plants has always been important to collectors. Unfortunately, no international system has yet successfully designed and implemented a system that provides for an effective legal protection of traditional knowledge holders at the international level.

A discussion paper 'Traditional Knowledge and Intellectual Property: Issues and options surrounding the protection of traditional knowledge' written by Carlos M Correa, of the University of Buenos Aires gives an excellent basis to this important debate. The protection under intellectual property rights (IPRs) of traditional and indigenous knowledge (TK) has received growing attention since the adoption of the Convention on Biological Diversity in 1992. Numerous contributions by academics, NGOs and governments have considered the need to provide some form of protection to TK. However, significant divergences exist as to whether IPRs should be applied and which would be the rationale and modalities of protection. It is important to understand the scope of TK, which includes its widespread use in TM and agriculture.

Professor Correa rightly feels that it is premature to promote international IPR-type standards for TK protection at present and suggests global rules to prevent misappropriation of TK. He also suggests various ways in which Overseas Development Assistance can be used to clarify and improve the present situation[176].

---

175 The Protection of Traditional Knowledge under Intellectual Property Law (2000), EIPR, p. 255.

176 Correa C.M. Traditional Knowledge and Intellectual Property: Issues and options surrounding the protection of traditional knowledge - A Discussion Paper commissioned by The Quaker United Nations Office (QUNO), Geneva2001, with financial assistance from the Rockefeller Foundation.

The field of intellectual property rights is rapidly changing and laws vary from country to country. American Association for the Advancement of Science (AAAS) has published a useful handbook to provide an accurate summary of TK, intellectual property concepts and options. Generally, all options are subject to respective national laws and legislation. AAAS handbook gives a detailed yet simple account of TK and IPR issues starting from the definition, scope, and concerns. It covers all the possible Intellectual Property Protection Options for Traditional Knowledge Holders including: Patents, Petty Patent Models, Plant Patents, Plant Variety Certificates, Traditional Knowledge Registries, Trade Secrets, Trademarks, Geographical Indicators, Prior Art and Defensive Disclosure, Prior Informed Consent, *Sui Generis* Protection Systems, Access and Benefit-Sharing. It also discusses important issues related to documenting TK, locating and identifying TK, identifying who holds the knowledge, identifying IP options, etc. with lot of examples[177]. Another document of AAAS provides important debate in reference to TK and globalized biopiracy[178].

Currently, some 95% of patents in the world are held in developed countries. International patent law and most national conventional patent law protection requirements of novelty and inventive steps do not seem to be applicable to traditional knowledge and biodiversity. For example, there is no act under patent law,\ which could be used to protect the non-medication traditional therapies, such as

[177] Stephen H. and Justin V. July 2003, Traditional Knowledge and Intellectual Property: A Handbook on Issues and Options for Traditional Knowledge Holders in Protecting their Intellectual Property and Maintaining Biological Diversity American Association for the Advancement of Science (AAAS), Washington, DC.

[178] Stephen H, Intellectual Property and Traditional Ecological Knowledge: Institutionally Globalized Biopiracy? Professional Ethics Report, 2002; 3(XV), 1-8.

manual therapies and spiritual therapies. Because of the lack of database and the same medicinal plants growing and being used in various countries and continents, it is very difficult to identify the founder. The great traditions like Ayurveda provide a rich information source. For instance, over 5000 herbo-mineral formulations[179] with rationale are provided by the traditional Ayurvedic system of medicine and would need protection. The existing conventional patent law can protect pharmaceutical products. However, herbal medicines and herbal products are quite different from chemical drugs. They are very difficult to be protected by the existing patent law[180].

Professor Gerry Bodeker has given an extensive review of the whole issue and has suggested new IPR models for the protection of traditional knowledge: Changing IPR law; Certificates of origin; Transforming traditional knowledge into trade secrets; Local innovations databases. India has the examples of the National TK Database (Traditional Knowledge Digital Library-TKDL) to Establish Prior Art on Indian Medicinal Heritage and the International Database to Establish Prior Art on TK Globally. He has also suggested some *sue generis* models for an equitable future. There is another effort of FRLHT where women farmers become stakeholders of a public company that undertakes organized cultivation and value addition activities[181]. This effort serves many objectives. First, it empowers poor rural

---

[179] Paranjape P. Traditional Ayurvedic Formulations, 2003, Chaukhamba Prakashan, Varanasi, India.

[180] Zhang Xiaorui. Traditional Medicine and Its Knowledge, UNCTAD Expert Meeting on "Systems and National Experiences for Protecting Traditional Knowledge, Innovations and Practices" UNCTAD, United Nations Palais des Nations, Geneva 30 October 2000.

[181] Darshan Shankar, Foundation for Revitalization of Local Health Traditions, Banglore.

women farmers by providing newer ways of income generation. Secondly, it helps in optimal use of traditional medicine knowledge available with the local communities. Thirdly, it provides quality herbal material to industries and other bulk users and helps in replacing cultivated sources in place of wildly collected herbal materials.

Despite the trend for the herbal sector to develop products based on TK and to rely on market edge and competitive forces as a means of gaining market share and profit, there has been a growing trend of herbal or natural products companies specializing in the medicinal applications of plant extracts to seek patents for application of Traditional Medicine Knowledge (TMK). Some such examples include: an appetite suppressant of the San People of the Kalahari; a traditionally-based AIDS medicine in South Africa; a famous case of Andean Maca and Indian example of Jeevani plant of Kani tribes of Kerala from South India for benefit sharing between the communities and herbal industry[182]. Collaborating with traditional healers remains a valid method for the identification of potential lead compounds for novel pharmaceuticals. However, the knowledge of these traditional healers is rapidly being lost. Historic herbal texts provide a unique window to identify plants whose specific uses are no longer known. Buenz *et al.* have identified nine plants in the 17th century, which were documented as having medicinal properties but have not been researched[183]. Such efforts may help to identify candidate specimens deserving further pharmacological study, yet they raise important issues related to IPR.

The international view on this issue is reflected in the June 2002 report in *Science.* The U.S. plans to limit the future

[182] P. Pushpangadan, CSIR India initiative that led to UNDP award 2003.

[183] Buenz E.J. Bioprospecting Rumphius's Ambonese Herbal: Volume I. Journal of Ethnopharmacology 2005; 96(1-2) 57-70.

patent rights of all foreign recipients of government grants and contracts to the awardee's own country and to have the U.S. National Institutes of Health retain the rights elsewhere. The *Science* report notes that this impacts immediately on NIH-funded research in Australia which led to discovery of two cytokines that can boost the immune system of cancer patients, and which are now marketed by companies such as Amgen and Schering-Plough and have generated revenues of more than $1.5 billion a year in U.S. sales. Australian scientists have lodged formal protests. The U.S. view is that such a move is in "the best interests of U.S. citizens" by making sure that they benefit fully from all NIH-funded research. From the perspective of TK, this will call into question the substance of the benefit sharing arrangements in the many inter-country agreements of NIH's National Cancer Institute[184].

IP protection for traditional medicines has multiple and diverse objectives. However, its priorities are often not clear and may confront with strategies and the prioritization of objectives. The differences in stakeholders' concepts on ownership of knowledge add to the problem. The policymakers should address these multiple, multi-layered issues and questions, and try to develop a range of solutions to address and balance the various objectives and interests[185]. One project that has been proposed to develop such information is the Global IP, Benefit Sharing and Traditional Medicine Database. It is being developed as a component of the Global Information Hub on Integrated Medicine from the work of the Commonwealth Working Group (CWG) on Traditional and Complementary Health

[184] Jocelyn Kaiser, N.I.H. to Limit Scope of Foreign Patents, Science, 2002, 296, 2316.

[185] Timmermans K. Intellectual property rights and traditional medicine: policy dilemmas at the interface. Soc Sci Med. 2003;57(4):745-56.

Systems, now directed by the Malaysian Ministry of Health. This Information Hub is planning to create a network of legal centers, scholars and NGOs working together to develop a comprehensive legislative and policy review, information resource and exchange on issues pertaining to IP rights over traditional medical knowledge and the use of medicinal plants[186].

The complexity of the situation outlined above brings us inevitably to consider some *sui generis* options to protect TK and its legitimate owners from exploitation. By very definition such laws do not fit within existing frame of law and such class does not belong to any taxonomic class[187]. However, *sui generis* evolved exactly to accommodate such impasse.

Markets, Business and Trade

The IP/TK debate has reached new levels of serious review and new prospects for TK protection since the Doha meeting of November 2001 and the resulting process for the harmonization of TRIPS and Convention on Biological Diversity. The growth of the herbal sector and the constant demand for new and saleable traditional medical products is new in the field of IP and traditional medical knowledge. This trend will clearly grow and should become a primary focus of IPR development. There is a need for the herbal industry to become more proactive and responsive to this dimension. The herbal and traditional medicine industry should voluntarily develop in-house industry standards that are based on ethical practices and are overseen jointly by industry-government-NGO-indigenous monitoring groups.

---

[186] Gerard Bodeker, Traditional (i.e. Indigenous) and Complementary Medicine in the Commonwealth: New Partnerships Planned With the Formal Health Sector, Journal of Alternative & Complementary Medicine 1999; 5, 97.

[187] http://en.wikipedia.org/wiki/Sui_generis.

To provide new models for development, information needs to be gathered on current practices. This in turns needs to be analyzed according to principles of best practice in benefit sharing and IPR. *Sui generis* systems alone may or may not be the way forward although, it offers a unique local means of protecting TM that works for the local context. At the same time, it is at risk of being un-enforceable outside of the country or region of origin and hence creating vulnerability to the biopiracy that it is expected to prevent. For *sui generis* systems to work, there is need to be reciprocity among countries to respect one another's local *sui generis* regimes. Although, it would seem somewhat difficult in the current international IP political environment, such developments require backing and enforcement within the context of national and international IPR regimes. This would require WIPO, the CBD and the WTO to coordinate their policies and legal instruments in partnership with TK holders as well as with conventional stakeholders such as governments and industry. If this can be achieved, the health benefits offered to the world through the globalization of traditional medical knowledge also stand to benefit communities and countries in terms of economic development and the growth of national pride in the preservation of culture through the principles of fair trade[188].

At the first Global Knowledge Conference in Toronto in 1997, political leaders and civil society representatives from developing countries endorsed the vision of the World Bank to become a "Knowledge Bank" that intermediates ideas as well as resources. In 2004, the World Bank published a book entitled *Indigenous Knowledge – Local Pathways to Global Development* that was formally launched

[188] Bodeker. G. Traditional Medical Knowledge, Intellectual Property Rights & Benefit Sharing. Cardozo Journal of Int'l & Comp. Law, 2003; 11:785-814.

in October 2004 in Tanzania. The partnership between the World Bank and the Global Research Alliance (GRA) in the domain of indigenous knowledge is expected to contribute to advanced research and development without compromising the interests of indigenous communities.

Biodiversity

Fifth meeting of Global Forum for Bioethics in Research held at Paris in April 2004 dealt in detail with issues related to Equity and Intellectual Property. One related presentation by Professor Anil Gupta highlights the inadequacies in the technical competence and infrastructural capabilities of most of the developing countries. An international registry administered electronically by WIPO might provide the most effective tool for meeting the aspirations of grassroots innovators and traditional knowledge holders. This registry should help accomplish a golden triangle of rewarding creativity by linking innovation, investment and enterprise around the globe. Without a system of protection of knowledge globally, incentives for disclosure and dissemination cannot be provided to the holders of valuable traditional knowledge about biological and genetic resources as well as other resources. If exploitation of knowledge has to be controlled, we may need online intellectual property rights administration[189]. The symbiotic relation between biodiversity and drug discovery involving natural product drug discovery is well reviewed by Geoffrey A. Cordell, University of Illinois at Chicago[190].

---

[189] Gupta A.K. IP for Traditional knowledge on-line: Recognizing, Respecting and Rewarding Creativity and Innovation at Grassroots. Invited Paper presented at the Second WIPO International Conference on Electronic Commerce and Intellectual Property, Geneva, 19-21 September, 2001.

[190] Cordell G.A. Biodiversity and drug discovery - a symbiotic relationship. Phytochemistry 2000; 55(6), 463-480.

A 'Banglore Declaration[191] July 2004' made during a workshop in India deliberated in detail issues related to medicinal plants, biodiversity, cultivation, R&D, IPR, documentation, TM etc. This document provides a good vision statement that stresses the importance of providing sustainable livelihood opportunities to small and medium farmers and the rural poor in the region through organic cultivation systems and sustainably managed collection; to provide affordable healthcare options in the form of high quality traditional medicines to domestic markets in the region; to progressively build regional brands in the global markets, using this as a means to tap the lucrative and fast growing markets for products and services in the healthcare, neutraceuticals, health foods, fragrances, dyes and cosmetics business segments; aggressive marketing of products while safeguarding the resource base of the raw products.

Many traditional medicines use natural materials including plant and animal origin that may cause serious threat to biodiversity. For instance Tiger bone has been used as a treatment for rheumatism and related ailments for thousands of years in traditional Asian medicine. In the early 1990s, it became evident that medicinal trade in Tiger bone threatened to drive the already endangered Tiger to extinction in the wild. The importance of this threat was documented in the 1994 TRAFFIC report, Killed For A Cure: A Review of the Worldwide Trade in Tiger Bone[192]. Not just tigers but the whole range of wild animals or their

---

[191] Workshop on Medicinal Herbs & Plants: Scope for Diversified and Sustainable Extraction, Funded by Common Fund for Commodities (CFC) Amsterdam in collaboration with Bio Centre and Food & Agriculture Organization, Rome held at Banglore India during July 22 – 26, 2004.

[192] Michael't Sas-Rolfes, Who Will Save the Wild Tiger?, PERC Policy Series, Issue Number PS-12, February 1998.

materials are used in TM - Rhino, Deer, Elephants, and many such are under threat. It is same with medicinal plants and marine materials. Medicinal plants classified as endangered species in the red book such as *Taxus Spp, Swartia Spp.* and many others are being prohibited for commercial collection from their habitats. For instance corals, deer horns etc are part of important Ayurvedic medicines and are prohibited for use in medicines. While their use was previously limited to use for local communities, the increasing market demands are putting pressure on collectors and even as traders wooing them add to this problem. In India, the Department of Environment and Forest recently raided Ayurvedic manufacturers and filed legal cases for violating the biodiversity conservation regulations. This has created uproar and has resulted in unavailability of such medicine. This issue needs to be properly discussed with indigenous people and has to be resolved with out causing harm to either of the interests. Recently a National Seminar addressing issues related to globalization and herbal products organized at Mumbai gives a very representative Declaration[193] "The Indian subcontinent harbors one of the richest biodiversity of medicinal plants and the therapeutic benefits of these plants have been well documented in various treatise. Though these medicinal plants have documented history of centuries of therapeutic usage, these applications need validation applying the modern scientific approach. These validations need to address issues arising due to modern agricultural practices and mass collection procedures. The issues of safety, efficacy and stability of herbal formulations need to be resolved. Clinical trials need to be initiated keeping in view the traditional methods of diagnosis and prescription

[193] National Seminar On Globalising Ayurvedic And Herbal Products; Challenges And Strategies 4-5, February 2005, Renaissance Convention Centre, Powai, Mumbai, India.

with collaborative participation of experts from modern medicine. Well-designed training modules and courses need to be initiated to develop trained human resources for dealing with inter-disciplinary exercises of evaluations and investigations. Special training programs in Good Agricultural and Collection Practices for farmers need to be initiated with an aim to ensure consistent raw material quality. Regulatory schedules must be suitably amended to incorporate definition and standards for statistically proven plant based medicinal substances. Standardization programs must involve cultivation of medicinal plants, Raw material sourcing (vendor qualifications), raw material storage and transport, raw material processing, safety, efficacy and stability of formulation, limits of contaminants and adulterants and the patient information dossiers."

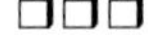

Part II : Development

6 Safety and Regulatory Issues

Safety is a primary concern regarding traditional and complementary therapies. There are two aspects of safety evaluations. First, to ensure that the right quality of material and apt possesses are used from sourcing to marketing; and second, there is no contamination, adulteration or spiking. Few studies have reported adulteration with steroids in some traditional Chinese dermatological preparations. In an analysis of Chinese herbal creams prescribed for dermatological conditions, Keane et al. found that eight of eleven creams analyzed contained steroids[194]. Spiking with corticostreoinds has been observed in some market preparations claimed to be useful in the treatment of arthritis and asthma[195]. Recently, Saper *et al.* from Harvard Medical School have reported heavy metal content of Ayurvedic herbal preparations and have recommended mandatory toxic heavy metal testing[196]. There have been few reports of heavy metal toxicity following traditional medicine use[197,198]. Such studies are

194 Keane FM. Analysis of Chinese herbal creams prescribed for dermatological conditions BMJ 1999;318:563-564.

195 Chopra A. & Doiphode V. Medical Clinics of North America 2002; 86:75-89.

196 Saper R.B. *et. al.,* Heavy metal content of Ayurvedic herbal medicinal preparations.JAMA 2004, 292 (23); 2868-2873.

197 Ernst E. Heavy metals in traditional Indian remedies. Eur J Clin Pharmacol. 2002; 57(12): 891-6.

198 Caldas ED, Machado LL. Cadmium, mercury and lead in medicinal herbs in Brazil. Food Chem Toxicol. 2004;42(4):599-603.

important and needed, however they are more related to the quality control failures of the mass manufacturing activities. Often they are wrongly used to limit the use of TM. In reality, such a QC failure should not be considered as a general negative notion to create a bias against TM. We certainly need effective QC and regulation of herbal medicines, without limiting public access to these preparations and ensuring public interest and constituting restrictive trade practice.

Traditionally, Ayurveda uses many metals in therapeutics but it is only after a due purification processes strictly followed in accordance with authentic traditional methods. Such traditional metal preparations (generally called as *Bhasma* and wrongly perceived as oxides are actually organometallic complexes) must qualify three main properties: ultrafine particle size that floats on water and one should not be able to recover metal back from the such preparations. Some of the recent studies have observed presence of nanoparticles in such traditional metallic preparations[199]. Most of the traditional methods for preparation of herbomineral complexes are very tedious and lengthy. Mass scale commercial production often tends to process a compromise that results adversely on its quality. This is the main reason of such heavy metal contaminations. What is more worrying is the fact that traditional preparations such as *mahasudarshan churna and bala guti* where metals are not the part of official formulation have shown high amount of toxic heavy metals. This is certainly a failure of the quality assurance system and a case of bad manufacturing processes. This is equally a failure of the regulatory system particularly the Indian that has not yet been able to evolve and enforce effective quality control

[199] Ashok Vaidya, 2003, Bhavans SPARC, Juhu, Mumbai (unpublished work) and Shastri M., 2004, Nano materials Group, National Chemical Laboratory, Pune India (unpublished work).

and safety assurance of herbal medicines. Government of India has released GMPs herbal medicines that need to be implemented strictly. It will be unfair to convey a general message against Ayurvedic or such traditional herbal medicines. In fact, Ayurveda or TM has nothing to do with it[200].

Research should consider best evidence for safety, including evidence for adverse effects from treatments and inappropriate applications of traditional therapies. Post-marketing surveillance studies can provide information on adverse effects of botanical herbal preparations. Pharmacognostic and pharmacological research can provide information on the quality, efficacy, safety or toxicity of botanical/herbal medicinal preparations[201]. More broadly, in addressing safety in herbal medicines, a basic question is 'safe with respect to what'? Research has found that in the US, 51% of FDA-approved drugs have serious adverse effects not detected prior to their approval. 1.5 million people are sufficiently injured by prescription drugs annually that they require hospitalization. Once in hospital, the problem may be compounded. The incidence of serious and fatal adverse drug reactions (ADRs) in US hospitals is now ranked as between the fourth and the sixth leading cause of death in the United States, following next after heart disease, cancer, pulmonary disease and accidents[202]. Thus, the safety of and risks associated with medical interventions is an issue across all categories of health care.

---

[200] Patwardhan *et.al.*, 2005. Heavy Metals and Ayurveda, Current Science, 88 (11).

[201] Warude D., Patwardhan B., Botanicals: Quality and regulatory issues.. J. of Scientific & Industrial Research, 2005 (In Press)

[202] Lazarou J, *et.al.*, Incidence of adverse drug reactions in hospitalized patients: A meta-analysis of prospective studies. JAMA 1998; 279:1200-5.

Safety must be the starting point in drug development strategies for herbal medicines. While most of the published research on herbal medicine is pharmacological, WHO's 1993 Guidelines on the Evaluation of Herbal Medicines considers that clinical evaluation is ethical where drugs have long been in traditional use. The Council for Scientific and Industrial Research of Government of India along with the Indian Council for Medical Research has offered a model for the clinical evaluation of herbal medicines[203]. This is being followed for the ongoing major herbal drug development program under the New Millennium Indian Technology Initiative has adopted the Reverse Pharmacology Approach (see Innovation and Drug Discovery section for details) and advocates adherence to mandatory requirements for clinical testing of any traditional preparation: Heavy metals, Pesticides, Microbial (pathogenic) load, are within the WHO prescribed limits and basic safety established in experimental animals using OECD guidelines[204].

Similarly, the dietary supplements that may come from out side of TM, have also been confronted with adverse events. Palmer *et al.* have reported in the observational study that Dietary supplements are associated with adverse events that include all levels of severity, organ systems, and age groups. Associations between adverse events and ingredients are difficult to verify if a product has more than one ingredient, and because of incomplete information systems[205]. In Nature Reviews Drug Discovery, Engel & Straus have discussed the regulatory framework for

---

[203] ICMR Guidelines for Clinical Trials in India, 2003.

[204] CSIR-NMITLI Government of India, Herbal Drug Development project, Clinical guidelines, 2003.

[205] Palmer M.E. *et. al.*, Adverse events associated with dietary supplements: an observational study. Lancet 2003; 361: 101–06

dietary supplements and drugs, outlined the challenges of evaluating dietary supplements for safety and clinical effectiveness, and also describe the evolving drug model for botanicals[206].

Global Forum on Safety of Herbal and Traditional Medicine report[207] has covered the status of regulation of complementary medicine in Australia and comparative examples from Africa and Bangladesh. Safety evaluation, which incorporates quality procedures, was identified as another point of focus. Clear evidence for the non-utilization of plants known to contain certain compounds producing deleterious effects has been exemplified via data and information on the dangers of ingesting pyrrolizidine alkaloids.

The Medicine and Healthcare Products Regulatory Agency of UK (MHRA) has produced a list of frequently asked questions and answers about the safety and quality of traditional Chinese medicines. According to MHRA there are some TCM products on the UK market that may be manufactured to low quality standards and may be deliberately adulterated or accidentally contaminated with toxic or illegal ingredients. These products do pose a direct risk to public health and it is not currently possible to distinguish between these products and TCMs that are made to acceptable safety and quality standards. The shortfall in quality standards may not be necessarily dangerous (except in cases of heavy metal, pesticide, pathogens or other such contaminations), but there is an element of risk. The risks vary widely, depending on the ingredients and how they are used. The former Medicines Control Agency informed the public in 2001 via the general media of the advice given

---

[206] Engel L. & Straus E., Nature Reviews Drug Discovery 2002, 1, 229 –237.

[207] Noller B.N., Global Forum on Safety of Herbal and Traditional Medicine: July 7, 2001, Gold Coast, Australia.

by the Committee on the Safety of Medicines (CSM) that it was not possible to give the public assurances as to the safety and quality of TCMs on the UK market. Since then the Agency (now the MHRA) has continued to find examples of illegal and dangerous TCMs being supplied in the UK and consumers should be alerted to the continuing problem. Recent samples of TCMs found on the UK, which pose a risk to public health, have contained mercury, heavy metals and toxic herbal ingredients.

The rising use of TM/CAM by the Australian public has also raised the critical issue of safety. Safety is assumed and rarely questioned. There is a general belief (also found in many other communities) that herbal or natural medicines are safe, which is obviously both simplistic and untrue. Yet, an Australian survey of 3027 people in 2000 showed that 90% of users of CAM (especially the elderly) considered the products safe, compared with 65% of non-users. The widespread availability of complementary medicines through health food stores and supermarkets, and the infrequency of litigation against CAM practitioners, has been suggested as evidence of safety. However, these need not be appropriate measures of safety. It is important to realize that any therapy has the potential to cause harm, and that any pharmacologically active product is likely to have adverse effects. The critical issue in assessing merit of any therapy is its risk to benefit. In modern medicine such therapeutic index outlining the number of individuals experiencing an adverse event versus the number of people achieving a benefit is fairly well studied and documented. The TM/CAM therapies and products need more rigorous assessment, systematic pharmacovigilance and till such time it is achieved satisfactorily, the clinicians should have a definite plan for understanding and valuing safety issues[208].

[208] Myers S. P. and Cheras P. A. The other side of the coin. MJA 2004; 181: 222–225

Herb-Drug interaction is a growing concern in TM. Single or multiple botanicals are bound to contain several chemical ingredients. Some of these chemicals are directly responsible for therapeutic activity, some are responsible for balancing the toxicity, some are required as carriers and some could be harmful as well. However, if the preparations are the result of traditional practices and continued use, the harmful part of it may be considered as low. However, in the modern world, when there are many other options available, there are many occasions when TM and modern medicine are used together. This opens a new dimension of herb-drug interaction. As such there are very few studies on this subject, however, available data certainly indicates seriousness and importance of herb-drug interactions[209]. Ginkgo: Causes bleeding when used with warfarin; causes raised blood pressure when used with a thiazide diuretic. Ginseng lowers blood concentrations of alcohol and warfarin; induces mania when used with phenelzine. Garlic lowers blood concentration of warfarin; changes the pharmacokinetics of paracetamol; causes hypoglycaemia when used with chlorpropamide. St John's wort[210] lowers blood concentrations of cyclosporin, amitriptyline, digoxin, indinavir, warfarin, phenprocoumon and theophylline; causes intermenstrual bleeding when used with oral contraceptives; causes mild serotonin syndrome when used with loperamide or selective serotonin reuptake inhibitors. These are just few studies that underline importance of better understanding of herb-herb or herb-drug interactions where more attention and research is urgently needed to ensure safety.

---

[209] Izzo A.A. and , Ernst E. Interactions between herbal medicines and prescribed drugs. Drugs 2002; 61: 2163-2175.

[210] Mills E. *et al.* Interaction of St John's wort with conventional drugs,. BMJ 2004, 329; 27-30.

Quality Control and Regulations

Traditional Medicine involves extensive use of botanicals and includes various steps starting from a passport data on raw materials, correct identification, pharmacognostic and physico-chemical quality standardization, safety and preclinical pharmacology (acute, sub-acute and choric toxicity studies), clinical pharmacology (pharmacokinetics and pharmacodynamics) and randomized controlled clinical trials (Phase I to Phase IV). While traditional health systems in developing countries have typically been the primary health service of rural communities and the poorest levels of society, there is now increasing reliance on traditional health care by urban populations as well[211]. In Africa, for instance, the rapid rate of urbanization is changing the face of traditional medicine. Where previously, the village herbalist or healer would provide services and would draw on nearby forests and fields for herbs, urban markets have many herb sellers, each giving advice and many selling both raw plant material and preparations that they have produced themselves. Almost similar situation exists in many parts including India where still main sources of herbs are coming from nature and not through planned cultivations. Quality control is a challenge under these circumstances.

Addressing quality control and standardization is very vital and needs broader consideration. The dynamic process of evolution could have altered and affected the identity and structure of natural materials. For commercialization, correct identification and supply of raw material to avoid adulteration has become a challenge. Additionally, some botanical species might have been extinct or may have

[211] Cunningham, A.B., 1993, African Medicinal Plants: Setting priorities at the interface between conservation and primary health care. People and Plants working paper. UNESCO 1993 Division of Ecological Sciences, Paris.

undergone change due to time and environmental factors. Standardization of botanicals and medicines is required differently, although one cannot readily apply the typical modern pharmaceutical pharmacopoeial standards. The concept of active markers in the process of standardization needs a flexible approach in favor of the very complex nature of these materials.

Recently, many international authorities and agencies including the World Health Organization[212], European Scientific Cooperation of Phytomedicine[213], US Agency for Health Care Policy and Research[214], European Pharmacopoeia Commission, Department of Health UK[215], Commonwealth of Australia[216], Department of Indian System of Medicine have started creating new mechanisms to induce and regulate quality control and standardization of botanical medicine. European Medicine Evaluation Agency has prepared proposal for directive from the European Commission for the Traditional Medicinal Products[217]. National Reference Centre for African Traditional Medicines: A South African Model made by

---

[212] General Guidelines for Methodologies on research and evaluation of Traditional Medicine In: World Health Organization, Geneva, WHO/EDM/TRM/2000.1. (2000). P 1-73.

[213] Note for guidance on Quality of Herbal Medicinal Products In: European Agency for the evaluation of Medicinal Products: EMEA/CVMP/814/00, (2001).

[214] Draft guidance for Industry on Botanical drug products In: U.S Department of Health and Human services, Food and Drug Administration and Center of drug evaluation and research: August 2000.

[215] Department of Health UK, Regulation of herbal medicine and acupuncture, Proposals for statutory regulation, March 2004.

[216] Expert Committee on Complementary Medicines in the Health System Report to the Parliamentary Secretary to the Minister for Health and Ageing September 2003.

[217] The Draft EC Proposal for a Directive on Traditional Medicines Keller Konstantin Chair of the Herbal Medicinal Products Working Group European Medicines Evaluation Agency, London.

Department of Health Medical Research Council, Council for Scientific and Industrial Research presents a good example. While regulation of traditional medicines remains a challenge, progress has been made in South Africa by the National Department of Health to provide for a regulatory framework to register, regulate and control African Health Practitioners. The proposed Traditional Healers Bill will establish a traditional Healers' Council once it becomes law. There is a need for a comprehensive review and development of policy and legislation pertaining to traditional health care, incorporating standards of accreditation, training and research. A botanical drug or a preparation thereof is now regarded as one active substance in its entirety whether or not the constituents with therapeutic activity are known. This will be a major step in development of new generation standardized botanical medicines.

The regulatory and legal situation regarding TM and herbal preparations varies from country to country. In some, herbal medicines are well established, whereas in others they are regarded as food where therapeutic claims are not allowed. Recently, De Smet has discussed many issues related to regulatory standards for herbal medicines in Europe[218]. Developing countries, however, often have a great number of traditionally used herbal medicines and much folk-knowledge about them, but have often inadequate legislative criteria to establish them as part of the drug legislation. For the classification of herbal or traditional medicinal products, factors applied in regulatory systems include: mention in traditional classic books as in case of Auyuvedic medicines in India[219]. Additionally,

[218] DeSmet Peter A.G.M., Herbal medicine in Europe – Relaxing regulatory standards. N. Engl. J. Med., March 2005, 352;12:1176-78.

[219] FDA Schedule on Ayurvedaaaic Medicines, Government of India.

description in pharmacopoeia monograph, prescription status, claim of a therapeutic effect, scheduled or regulated ingredients or substances, or periods of use are also considered. Some countries draw a distinction between officially approved products and officially recognized products, by which the latter products can be marketed without scientific assessment by the authority. Dr. Xiaorui Zhang of Traditional Medicine Program of WHO has taken an excellent worldwide overview of regulatory status of TM.

The WHO has published many official and nonofficial documents on TM related subjects including WHO Monographs on selected medicinal plants[220]. Global definitions of botanical products are being developed by international cooperation and a new perspective of standardization, validation, safety and efficacy of botanical medicines is evolving, which is a good sign[221]. Multi-component botanical formulations can be standardized with newer techniques such as DNA fingerprinting[222], High Pressure Thin Layer Chromatography, hyphenated techniques such as Liquid Chromatography-Mass Spectroscopy. In-house monographs need to be evolved and critically followed. For example, a multi-component botanical formulation (Artrex) designed for the treatment of arthritis contains four botanicals and all ingredients, their respective extracts and the formulation are standardized using HPLC and HPTLC fingerprint profiles with known markers. This formulation has been granted a US Patent[223]

---

[220] WHO Monographs on selected medicinal plants Volume I and II, 1996, 97.

[221] Warude D., Patwardhan B., Botanicals: Quality and regulatory issues.. J. of Scientific & Industrial Research, April 2005 (In Press).

[222] Joshi K. *et. al.*, Molecular markers in Herbal Drug Technology, Current Science, 2004, 87(2) 159-165.

[223] Patwardhan B. A method of treating musculoskeletal disease and a novel composition therefor. United States Patent No. 5,494,668, February 1996.

and is commercially available in India and few other countries. Pre-clinical studies on Ayurvedic medicines are more important for validating drug safety resulting from new procedures or extractions are used during its preparation. The value of animal testing to establish safety and toxicity is not so critical if the botanicals are used in traditional forms. Suitable animal models help in understanding the mechanism of action or pharmacodynamics of medicines, however, no good animal models exist for some human diseases.

The basis of traditional medicine is its use for number of years and therefore its clinical existence comes as a priori assumption. However, for bringing more objectivity and also to confirm traditional claims, systematic clinical trials are necessary. In TM research, clinical experiences, observations or available data becomes a starting point. In conventional drug research it comes at the last. Thus, the drug discovery based on TM follows a 'Reverse Pharmacology' path[224]. Nevertheless, all the critical Pharmacopoeial tests such as dissolution time, microbial, pesticide and heavy metals contamination etc. must be in accordance with global standards. It is important to ensure that all the TM manufacture is in accordance with Current Good Manufacturing Procedures for herbal products[225,226].

---

[224] Vaidya A.D.B., Vaidya R.A., Nagaral S.I. Ayurveda and a different level of evidence: From Lord Macaulay to Lord Walton (1835-2001 AD), Journal of Association of Physicians India (JAPI), 2001; 49:534-537 and Approach Paper, New Millennium Indian Technology Leadership Initiative Herbal Drug Development Program, CSIR New Delhi, 2002.

[225] Good manufacturing practices: Supplementary guidelines for manufacture of Herbal Medicinal products In: WHO expert committee on specifications for pharmaceutical preparations. Thirty fourth report. Geneva, World Health Organization, 1996,Annex8 (WHO technical Series, no 863). P.134-139.

[226] Verpoorte R and Mukherjee P. GMP for Botanicals, businesshorizons.com, 2003.

There have been many concerns about quality standards and safety issues of herbal medicines[227]. The need for new regulations for TM and natural medicines has been frequently stressed and some such regulations are coming in force in different parts of the world[228,229].

Herbal Drug Development: Issues and Regulations

Herbal drug development includes various steps starting from a passport data on raw materials, correct identification, pharmacognostic and chemical quality standardization, safety and preclinical pharmacology, clinical pharmacology and randomized controlled clinical trials. Addressing standardization is very vital and needs broader consideration. Ayurvedic medicine was developed at times of limited access to technologically and variable norms of standardization. The dynamic process of evolution could alter and affect the identity and structure of natural materials. For commercialization, correct identification and supply of raw material to avoid adulteration has become a challenge. Additionally, some botanical species might have been extinct. Lastly, the properties of botanicals as recorded in classics may have undergone change due to time and environmental factors. Standardization of Ayurvedic botanicals and medicines is required although one cannot readily apply the typical modern pharmaceutical pharmacopoeial standards. The concept of active markers in the process of standardization needs a flexible approach in favor of the very complex nature of these materials.

---

[227] Straus S. Herbal Medicines – What's in the Bottle? NEJM 2002: 347(25);1997-1998.

[228] Legal Status of Traditional Medicine- A Worldwide Review, W.H.O. Geneva 2001.

[229] Marcus D and Grollman A. Botanical Medicines – The need for new regulations, NEJM 2002: 347(25); 2073-2076.

Recently, many international authorities and agencies including the World Health Organization[230], European Agency for the Evaluation of Medicinal Products and European Scientific Cooperation of Phytomedicine[231], US Agency for Health Care Policy and Research[232], European Pharmacopoeia Commission, Department of Indian System of Medicine have started creating new mechanisms to induce and regulate quality control and standardization of botanical medicine. For Ayurvedic medicine and other traditional medicines newer guidelines of standardization are required. A botanical drug or a preparation thereof is now regarded as one active substance in its entirety whether or not the constituents with therapeutic activity are known. This will be a major step in development of new generation standardized botanical medicines. The WHO has published official documents on medicinal plants and WHO Monographs on selected medicinal plants[233]. Global definitions of botanical products are being developed by international cooperation and a new perspective of standardization, validation, safety and efficacy of botanical medicines is evolving - and is a good sign. Multi-component botanical formulations can be standardized with newer techniques such as DNA fingerprinting, High Pressure Thin Layer Chromatography, Liquid chromatography-Mass Spectroscopy In-house monographs need to be evolved and critically followed. For example a multi-component

---

[230] General Guidelines for Methodologies on research and evaluation of Traditional Medicine In: World Health Organization, Geneva, WHO/EDM/TRM/2000.1. (2000). P 1-73.

[231] Note for guidance on Quality of Herbal Medicinal Products In: European Agency for the evaluation of Medicinal Products: EMEA/CVMP/814/00, (2001).

[232] Draft guidance for Industry on Botanical drug products In: U.S Department of Health and Human services, Food and Drug Administration and Center of drug evaluation and research: August 2000.

[233] WHO Monographs on selected medicinal plants Volume I and II, 1996, 97.

botanical formulation (Artrex) designed for the treatment of arthritis contains four botanicals and all ingredients, their respective extracts and the formulation are standardized using HPLC and HPTLC fingerprint profiles with known markers. This formulation has been granted a US Patent[234].

Regulatory Aspects for Quality

Consistency in composition and biological activity are essential requirements for the safe and effective use of therapeutic agents. Quality is the critical determinant of safety and efficacy of botanical medicines; however, botanical preparations rarely meet the quality standards. These difficulties may be due to problems in identifying correct plant, genetic variability, variable growing conditions, differences in harvesting procedures and processing of the materials and lack of information about therapeutically active principles. Use of chromatographic techniques and chemical marker assisted characterization of the botanicals does not ensure consistent biological activity or stability. Therefore, production of quality botanical medicines has become a challenge to regulatory authorities, scientific organizations and manufacturers. WHO, USFDA, European Scientific Cooperative on Phytomedicine (ESCOP) have published standard sets of guidelines to address the issues. Most of the botanical manufacturers of the world follow them for providing standardized botanical medicine. In India, about 9000 licensed firms manufacture traditional medicines with or without proper standardization. Indian manufacturers generally follow WHO standards for quality control. India needs its own parameters and standard sets of guidelines for quality control of Ayurvedic medicines. WHO defined

---

[234] Patwardhan B. A method of treating musculoskeletal disease and a novel composition therefor. United States Patent No. 5,494,668, February 1996.

standards for mycotoxin contamination in herbals; however, its incidence is higher in tropical and subtropical countries as harvesting conditions and temperature and moisture contents are conducive to fungal invasion and mycotoxin elaboration. Adulteration of market samples remains a major problem in domestic and export markets of Indian herbal products. Market botanicals are stored under undesirable conditions over the years and may have contamination or adulteration of other materials thereby adversely affect the efficacy and sometimes even add to toxicity. Lack of proper processing of the materials even by pharmaceutical firms contributes to decline of the herbal business and global promotion of Ayurveda. Availability of the desired genotype of the plant in the required quantity, free from toxic contaminants and with desired therapeutic activity has also become a critical issue. Government of India has promulgated GMP regulations for traditional systems of medicines to improve the quality and standard of Ayurvedic, Siddha and Unani drugs in pharmacies. New rules delineating essential infrastructure, manpower and quality control requirements came into force from July 23, 2000 and form part of the Drugs and Cosmetics Act, 1940. Standardization of herbal drugs is not just an analytical operation for identification and assay of active principles; rather, it comprises total information and controls to necessarily guarantee consistent composition of all herbals. A good example of this is a polyherbal formulation (Artrex) designed for the treatment of arthritis contains four botanicals. The formulation has been standardized using modern scientific tools and with known markers, which has been granted a US patent. Proven agroindustrial technologies should be applied for cultivation and processing of medicinal plants and manufacturing of herbal medicines. Indian herbal drug industry needs to ensure procurement of standardized authentic raw material free from toxic contaminants, improving processing technologies, conducting all operations under GMP compliance and maintenance of in-process quality control for manufacturing quality herbal products with proven therapeutic efficacy, safety and shelf-life. The licensed manufacturers of Ayurveda would have two years to comply with the regulations and to obtain GMP certification.

Policy Issues

Developed nations till now freely exploited natural resources from the third world and the developing countries. With the devastation being wreaked in the tropical rainforests and the resurgence in interest in recent years in the discovery of novel drugs from natural sources, particularly plants and marine organisms, the international scientific community has realized that the conservation of these global genetic resources and the indigenous knowledge associated with their use are of primary importance if their potential is to be fully explored. Efforts are initiated to achieve these goals through collaboration with, and fair and equitable compensation of, the scientists and communities of the genetically rich source countries. The signing of the United Nations Convention on Biological Diversity by nearly all of the World's nations has emphasized the need for the implementation of such policies.

Government of India too has expressed support and encouragement for the traditional medicine. A separate department for Indian Systems of Medicine and Homeopathy (ISM&H) now known as AYUSH (Ayurveda, Yoga, Unani, Siddha, Homoeopathy) was established in March 1995 to ameliorate the problems that indigenous systems face. Priorities include education, standardization of drugs, enhancement of availability of raw materials, research and development, information, communication and larger involvement of this type of medicine in the national system for delivering health care. The Central Council of Indian Medicine (CCIM) oversees teaching and training institutes while Central Council for Research in Ayurveda and Siddha (CCRAS) deals with interdisciplinary research. Some TIM products are being added into family welfare programs of the government under the World Bank project. These medicines are mainly for common diseases like anemia, edema during pregnancy, postpartum problems such as pain, uterine, and abdominal complications, difficulties with lactation, nutritional deficiencies and childhood diarrhea. The government has also established 10 new drug testing laboratories for traditional medicine and is upgrading existing laboratories to provide documented high quality evidence to licensing authorities for the safety and quality of herbal medicines. This replaces the earlier ad hoc system of testing that was considered unreliable. Randomized, controlled clinical trials of selected prescriptions for Indian systems of medicine have been initiated. These will demonstrate the safety and efficacy of the prescriptions and provide a basis for their international licensure as medicines rather than simply as food supplements The industry has not been able to grow and develop optimally during the last few decades. Largely the growth achieved is due to industry's own initiatives, in house research and development. A national organization: Ayurvedic Drugs Manufacturers' Association (ADMA) is taking a proactive role to improve quality and research that needs to be nurtured, stimulated and sustained by providing special funding or incentives. Preparation of formularies and pharmacopoeial standards has been attempted but a lot remains to be done.

❑❑❑

7 Quality Control and Standardization

Despite its existence and continued use over many centuries, and its popularity and extensive use during the last decade, traditional medicine has not been officially recognized in most countries. Consequently, education, training and research in this area have not been accorded due attention and support. The quantity and quality of the safety and efficacy data on traditional medicine are far from sufficient to meet the criteria needed to support its use world-wide. The reasons for the lack of research data are due to not only to health care policies, but also to a lack of adequate or accepted research methodology for evaluating traditional medicine[235].

The statement from General Guidelines for Methodologies on Research and Evaluation of Traditional Medicines (World Health Organization, 2000) highlights the need for consensuous in addressing the problems related to the quality of botanical drugs, which ultimately is a critical determinant of safety and efficacy of medicine. Further, the distribution and widespread sale of adulterated, misbranded, spurious botanical drug products and marked

[235] WHO General Guidelines for Methodologies on Research and Evaluation of Traditional Medicine, WHO/EDM/TRM/2000.

increase in misleading health claims of these products demands proper regulations on botanical medicine to protect public health[236]. Considering these two issues development of parameters for quality control standardization and regulatory norms for controlling the growing business of botanicals is a big task. Various regulatory authorities, research organizations and botanical drug manufacturers are constantly contributing to developing guiding principles addressing issues related to quality, safety and efficacy[237]. In this chapter we have highlighted problems associated with quality control of the botanicals and tried to guide a way towards a globally acceptable quality standard.

Challenges in Quality Control

Consistency in composition and biologic activity are essential requirements for the safe and effective use of therapeutic agents. However, botanical preparations rarely meet this standard. This may be due to several problems associated with botanical products, which starts right from procurement of raw botanicals to final packaging of the botanical drug product. Some of the challenges are incorrect identification of plants, genetic variability, variable growing conditions, differences in harvesting procedures and variable preparation and processing of the botanicals. These ultimately lead to batch-to-batch variation resulting in variable therapeutic response. Use of chemoprofiling assisted quality control can help in batch-to-batch consistency but does not ensure consistent pharmacologic activity or stability. Moreover, analyses of purportedly standardized preparations reveal that botanical products

---

[236] Marcus D M and Grollman A P, Botanical Medicines — The Need for new regulations, The New Engl J of Med 347(25) (2002) 2073-2076.

[237] Bhutani K K, Strategies for R& D in natural products for the new millennium, JPAS 2 (2000) 91-98.

often do not contain the amount of the compound stated on the label. Their potency may vary and their purity is suspect. Many herbal products contain undisclosed prescription or over-the-counter drugs and heavy metals. Saper *et al.,*[238] has recently proved presence of toxic heavy metals in some Asian proprietary herbal medicine. The USFDA and other investigators have reported presence of prescription drugs, including glyburide, sildenafil, colchicine, adrenal steroids, alprazolam, phenylbutazone, and fenfluramine, in products claiming to contain only natural ingredients[239]. Further, lack of reports on adverse effects of these drugs is also a growing challenge in marinating quality.

Factors Affecting Quality

Geographical variation: It has been well documented that geographical conditions affect the active constituents of the medicinal plant and hence their activity profiles. Provenance variation in camptothecin concentrations of *Camptotheca acuminata*[240], phenolic composition of *Hypericum androsaemum,* essential oil of Thyme (*Thymus serpyllum L.*), Indian geranium (*Pelargonium* sp.), mentha sp and various other species have been documented[241]. Also, many researchers have studied geographical variation at the genetic level. RAPD-based molecular markers have been found to be useful in differentiating different accessions of

---

[238] Saper RB, Kales SN, Paquin J, Burns MJ, Eisenberg DM, Davis RB, Phillips RS. Heavy metal content of Ayurvedic herbal medicine products. JAMA 2004;292(23):2868-73.

[239] Goldman P. Herbal medicine today and the roots of the modern pharmacology. Ann Intern Med 2001;135:594-600.

[240] Liu Z, Zhou G, Xu S. Provenance variation in camptothecin concentrations of Camptotheca acuminata grown in China. New Forests 24: 215–224, 2002.

[241] Verlet, N. Trends of the medicinal and aromatic plant sector in France. Acta Horticulturae 1992, 306, 169-175.

Taxus wallichiana, neem, *Juniperus communis* L., *Codonopsis pilosula, Allium schoenoprasum* L., *Andrographis paniculata* collected from different locations. Other DNA based markers like AFLP, RFLP, micro and minisatellites are also in practice. Therefore, selection of the correct plant material from appropriate geographical location for better therapeutic efficacy has become of prime concern.

Inter/intra species variation: Genotypic characterization of plant species and strains is useful as most plants, though belonging to the same genus and species, may show considerable variation between strains. A good example of this is the fraudulent adulteration of Chianti wines with inferior quality grapes. This is also the case with medicinal plants, where the amounts of active chemicals may vary from plant to plant. Herbal drugs are consumed in most developed nations in the form of ethno-therapeutics nutraceuticals or are used as the primary source of medicinal compounds or their intermediates. The varying drug content of different species of herbal plants has been a problem in the production of standardized herbal medicines, where a particular plant from a region can be linked to a specific drug content and thus have a therapeutic value assigned to it, even though similar plants from another region may not share the same levels of the drug. Factors such as soil, climate and adaptability dictate the viability of a particular species and subsequently its drug content[242]. In such cases, study of variations in the genetic composition of the plant, in addition to varying amounts of the active drug compound also becomes important.

Botanical materials and crude drugs: Usually therapeutic activity is assigned to a particular plant part, which is due

---

[242] WHO guidelines on good agricultural and collection practices (GACP) for medicinal plants, WHO, Geneva, 2003.

to the variation of active constituents in different parts of a plant. Gingerols content in ginger rhizome, withanolides content in ashwagandha roots, kutcoside in kutki rhizome, sennoside in senna leaves are some of the therapeutic markers present in particular plant parts. Quantitative estimation of these markers becomes necessary to prevent adulteration with similar morphological but inactive herbal material. This will also help in preventing tainting the crude drugs with substandard varieties. Further, roots and rhizomes are most susceptible for microbial and fungal contamination. Appropriate measures should be taken during pre and post harvesting operations of these materials.

Time of harvesting: Seasonal, spatial, and interspecific variation of quercetin in *Apocynum venetum* and *Poacynum hendersonii*, sinomenine in *Caulis Sinomenii* has been well documented. Volatile oil containing plants are the most susceptible for variation in oil content when collected at different times or seasons. Study on seasonal variation in the composition of the essential oil of sea fennel show that all compositions of the oil show fluctuations in their relative amounts throughout the period under study. Capsaicin, a neurone blocking agent and stimulant to prostaglandin production is present in higher concentrations in the summer fruits than in the autumn fruits of Capsicum minimum. Maximum production of artemisinin from *Artemisia annua L.* was more closely associated with the specific photoperiod than with a specific stage of plant development. Therefore, time of collection of a particular herb should be selected in such a way that the active constituents are at higher level. It also depends on the plant part to be used. Detailed information concerning the appropriate timing of harvest is often available in national pharmacopoeias, published standards, official monographs and major reference books. However, it is well known that the concentration of biologically active constituents varies with the stage of plant growth and development. This also applies to non-targeted toxic or poisonous indigenous plant ingredients. The best time for harvest (quality peak season/ time of day) should be determined according to the quality and quantity of biologically active constituents rather than the total vegetative yield of the targeted medicinal plant parts. During harvest, care should be taken to ensure that no foreign matter, weeds or toxic plants are mixed with the harvested medicinal plant materials. Medicinal plants should be harvested under the best possible conditions, avoiding dew, rain or exceptionally high humidity. If harvesting occurs in wet conditions, the harvested material should be transported immediately to an indoor drying facility to expedite drying so as to prevent any possible deleterious effects due to increased moisture levels, which otherwise promote microbial fermentation and mold.

Post Harvesting Practices

Drying: Drying of herbal drugs implies removal of sufficient amount of moisture so as to make them resistant to decomposition and growth of microorganisms. The process of drying varies depending upon the final material required. If the enzymetic action is to be encouraged slow drying at moderate temperature is necessary. When the enzymetic action is not desired then drying should be as fast as possible. Essential oil containing herbs are susceptible to loss of the aroma if not dried properly or if the oil is not distilled out immediately. Depending upon the climatic conditions the drying process varies. In suitable climate open-air shade drying is preferred for drugs like clove, cardamom, cinnamon. Sun drying is preferred for drying of senna leaves, ashwagandha roots, amla fruits. In both cases there is need for arrangements to cover the drug at night. Drying on papers spread on wooden framework is also preferred to increase rate of drying. Drying using artificial heat is more rapid than both of the above methods. Tray driers, hot water pipes, and hot air ovens are generally used for this purpose. These methods are specifically advantageous in helping to retain the color of flowers and leaves and fragrance of aromatic drugs. As a general rule, the flowers and leaves should be dried at a temperature within the range of 20-40 C; while drying of stem, bark, roots and rhizome is preferred at a temperature range 30-65 C. Other artificial methods like infrared devices, baking, indirect fire, lyophilization, and freeze-drying can also prevent the loss of active ingredients.

Processing: Specific post-harvest processing is required for some medicinal plant materials. This is essential to improve purity of the plant part being employed, to reduce drying time, to prevent damage from mold, other microorganisms and insects, and to detoxify indigenous toxins. Common specific processing practices include pre-selection, peeling the skins of roots and rhizomes, boiling in water, steaming, soaking, pickling, distillation, fumigation, roasting, natural fermentation, treatment with lime and chopping. Processing procedures involving the formation of certain shapes, bundling and special drying may also have an impact on the quality of the medicinal plant materials.

Packaging and storage: Processed medicinal plant materials should be packaged as quickly as possible to prevent deterioration of the product and to protect against unnecessary exposure to potential pest attacks and other sources of contamination. Continuous in-process quality control measures should be implemented to eliminate substandard materials, contaminants and foreign matter prior to and during the final stages of packaging. Processed medicinal plant materials should be packaged in clean, dry boxes, sacks, bags or other containers in accordance with standard operating procedures. Records should be kept of batch packaging, and should include the product name, place of origin, batch number, weight, assignment number and date. The records should be retained for a period of three years or as required by national and/or regional authorities. Storage of the herbal material should be at the controlled temperature and humidity. Whenever required and when possible, fresh medicinal plant materials should be stored at appropriate low temperatures, ideally at 2-8 C; frozen products should be stored at less than -20 C.

Routine Pharmacognosy: Most of the guidelines suggest routine pharmacognostic techniques as macroscopic and microscopic evaluation along with other techniques for quality control of the botanicals. Characterization using sensory organoleptic parameters such as color, odor, taste, and surface characteristics are studied in macroscopic evaluation. The size and shape of the plant part used is also taken into consideration. However, since these characteristics are judged subjectively and substitutes and adulterants may closely resemble the genuine material, it is often necessary to substantiate the findings by microscopy and/or physicochemical analysis. An examination by microscopy alone cannot always provide complete identification, though when used in association with other analytical methods it can frequently supply invaluable supporting evidence.

Chemical Fingerprinting

Thin layer chromatography (TLC) is the preferred method for herbal drug analysis. Various pharmacopoeias as American Herbal Pharmacopoeia (AHP), Chinese drug monographs and analysis, Pharmacopoeia of the People's Republic of China etc. still suggest TLC to provide characteristic fingerprints of herbs. TLC is used as an easier method of initial screening with a semi-quantitative evaluation together with other chromatographic techniques. TLC is advantageous as it is simple and can be employed for a multiple sample analysis. For each plate, more than 30 samples can be studied simultaneously. Advancements in automated sample application, pre-coated silica gel plates and video/densitometric scanning has revolutionized the field of planar chromatography leading to the development of so-called High Performance Thin Layer Chromatography (HPTLC). With the help of this technique, it is possible to get quantitative information about the marker compounds along with a qualitative evaluation. Forced-flow planar chromatography (FFPC), rotation planar chromatography (RPC), overpressured-layer chromatography (OPLC), and lectroplanar chromatography (EPC) are some of the recent advances in the field of planar chromatography and are quite helpful for quality control of herbal medicine. Further, parallel- and serially-coupled layers open up new vistas for the analysis of a large number of samples (up to 216) for high throughput screening and for the analysis of very complex matrices[243].

High-performance liquid chromatography (HPLC) can be used to analyze almost all the compounds in the herbal medicines. Over the past decades, HPLC has received extensive application in the analysis of herbal medicines where reversed-phase columns are the system of choice. For effective separation of the desired compounds various factors as different compositions of the mobile phases, their pH adjustment, pump pressures, etc need to be controlled. New techniques, such as micellar electrokinetic capillary chromatography (MECC), high-speed counter-current chromatography (HSCCC), low-pressure size-exclusion

---

[243] Nyiredy S, Progress in forced-flow planar chromatography J Chromatogr. A 2003, 1000: 985-99.

chromatography (SEC), reversed-phase ion pairing have been recently developed in the field of liquid chromatography[244]. These advancements have provided new opportunities for more efficient separation of single constituents from botanicals. Coupling HPLC with advanced detection systems like evaporative light scattering detection (ELSD) will further increase the signal-to-noise ratio. ELSD is an excellent detection method for analysis of non-chromophoric compounds. This new detector provides a possibility for the direct HPLC analysis of many pharmacologically active components in herbal medicines, since the response of ELSD depends on the size, shape, and number of elute particles unlike the UV detector, which relies on the analysis structure and/or chromophore of analytes.

Electrophoretic Methods

Capillary electrophoresis (CE) was introduced in the early 1980's as a powerful analytical and separation technique. It allows an efficient way to document the complexity of a sample and can handle virtually every kind of charged sample components ranging from simple inorganic ions to DNA. Thus, there was an obvious increase of electrophoretic methods, especially capillary electrophoresis, used in the analysis of herbal medicines. Most preferred techniques are capillary zone electrophoresis (CZE), capillary gel electrophoresis (CGE) and capillary isoelectric focusing (cIEF). CE is promising for the separation and analysis of active ingredients in herbal medicines, since it needs only small amounts of standards and can analyze samples rapidly with very good separation ability. Recently, several studies dealing with herbal medicines have been reported and two kinds of medicinal compounds, i.e.

---

[244] Lianga YZ, Xie P, Kelvin Chanc K. Quality control of herbal medicines J Chromtogr B, 812 (2004) 53–70.

alkaloids and flavonoids have been studied extensively. Mixtures of low-molecular weight compounds are most effectively separated using CE.

Molecular Fingerprinting

DNA-based molecular markers have proved their utility in fields like taxonomy, physiology, embryology, genetics, etc. As the science of plant genetics progressed, researchers have tried to explore these molecular marker techniques for their applications in commercially important plants such as food crops, horticultural plants, etc. and recently in pharmacognostic characterization of botanical medicine. DNA-based techniques have been widely used for authentication of plant species of medicinal importance. This is especially useful in case of those that are frequently substituted or adulterated with other species or varieties that are morphologically and/or phytochemically indistinguishable. Moreover, molecular marker assisted selection of desired chemotypes is also a valuable application of these techniques.

Toxic Contaminants

Over the past decade several adverse effects, sometimes life threatening, of botanical medicines has been reported. This has raised many questions regarding safety of botanicals. These botanical medicines may be contaminated with microorganisms, excessive or banned pesticides, heavy metals, chemical toxins, and radioactive substances etc[35]. In order to avoid these unsafe side effects, the causes of contamination must be well understood and eliminated from botanical medicines.

Microbial Contamination

Medicinal plants are associated with a broad variety of microbial contaminants, mainly bacteria and fungi. Although bacterial endospores and fungal spores can be regarded as the two dominating groups of contaminants associated with medicinal plants, a broad diversity of bacterial, fungal cells and viruses can be found either in or on the plant material. Among these microorganisms, pathogens may also occur and this fact particularly limits the utilization of these plants[245]. Microbial contamination has the potential to render plant material toxic, either by transforming the benign chemicals in the plant into harmful substances, or through the microbes' production of toxic compounds. For example, the moulding of sweet clover (*Melilotus officinalis*) causes a chemical transformation of clover's constituents and the resultant compounds can cause hemorrhaging. The potentially toxic effects of bacterial and fungal endotoxins such as *Escherichia coli* endotoxin and aflatoxin from A*spergillus* sp. are well known.

Mycotoxins are toxic metabolites produced by certain fungi that can infect and proliferate on various agricultural commodities in the field and/or during storage. Mycotoxins may exhibit various toxicological manifestations; some are teratogenic, mutagenic and/or carcinogenic in susceptible animal species and are associated with various diseases in domestic animals, livestock, and humans in many parts of the world[246]. The different mycotoxins of relevance to human health are aflatoxins, ochratoxins, zearalenone, fumonisins, and trichothecenes.

Relatively limited number of reports exists about the presence of pathogenic microorganisms that affect botanical products. Czech *et. al.*,[247] has screened a broad spectrum of

---

[245] Wolfgang K, Erich C and Brigitte K, Microbial Contamination of Medicinal Plants-A Review, Planta Med 68 2002 5-15.

[246] Molecular biology and natural toxins. Food and Drug Administration Compliance Program Guidance Manual, 7307.001, Ch. 7.

[247] Czech E, Wolfgang K and Koop B, Microbial status of commercially available medicinal herbal drugs-screening study, Planta Med 67 (2001) 263-269.

pathogens and indicator germs. It was shown that these microorganisms are rarely found with the exceptions of *Bacillus cereus* and *Clostridium perfringens*. However, these two are spore formers and usually do not appear in magnitudes representing a real toxicity potential. Studies have been conducted to determine the types of fungi and their toxins contaminating medicinal plants, processed and non-processed foods[248] and other materials of plant origin. The commonly encountered fungal species are found to be *Fusarium, Aspergillus, Penicillium, Mucor, Rhizopus, Absidia, Alternaria, Cladosporium* and *Trichoderma*[249,250,251,252,253]. Hitokoto *et. al.,*[254] have shown that moulds like *Aspergillus, Penicillium, Rhizopus, Mucor, Cladosporium* and *Aureobasidium* spp. can be found quite often in association with botanicals, but mycotoxin producers were only present around the level of 2%. On the contrary, Kumar *et. al.,*[255] has detected considerable risk levels of aflatoxins in several botanical medicinal samples of different taxa.

---

[248] Cirillo T, Ritieni A, Galvano F and Amodio C R, Natural occurrence of deoxynivalenol and fumonisins B1 and B2 in Italian marketed foodstuffs, Food Addit Contam 20(6) (2003) 566-571.

[249] Halt M, Moulds and mycotoxins in herb tea and medicinal plants, J Epidemiol 14(3) (1998) 269-274.

[250] Abeywickrama K, Bean G A, Cytotoxicity of Fusarium species mycotoxins and culture filtrates of Fusarium species isolated from the medicinal plant Tribulus terrestris to mammalian cells, Mycopathologia 120(3) 1992 189-193.

[251] Aziz H N, Youssef Y A, El-Fouly M Z and Moussa L A, Contamination of some common medicinal plant samples and spices by fungi and their mycotoxins. Bot Bull Acad Sin 39(4) (1998) 278-285.

[252] Blunden. G, Roch OG, Rogers DJ, *et. al.,* Mycotoxins in food, Med Lab Sci 48(4) (1991) 271-282.

[253] Vrabcheva T M, Mycotoxins in spices, Vopr Pitan 69(6) 2000 40-43.

[254] Hitokoto H, *et. al.,* Fungal contamination and mycotoxin detection of herbal drugs, Appl Environ Micro 36 (1978) 252-256.

[255] Kumar S, *et. al.,* Occurrence of aflatoxin in some liver curative herbal medicines, Letters in Applied Micro 17 (1993) 112-114.

Risk assessment of the microbial load of medicinal plants has become an important subject in the establishment of modern Hazard Analysis and Critical Control Point (HACCP) schemes. Various guidelines such as WHO, British Herbal Pharmacopoeia (BHP), Indian Herbal Pharmacopoeia, European Pharmacopoeia, ESCOP have issued special guidance for assessing microbial contaminations of both raw as well as processed botanicals. All these guidelines provide specific limits for the contaminants. These limits give due consideration to the level of treatment given to the material while processing. WHO Quality Control Methods for Medicinal Plant Materials mentions that the presence of aflatoxins can be hazardous to health if absorbed even in very small amounts and should therefore be determined after using suitable clean-up procedure. The document also contains the procedure for qualitative determination of aflatoxins B1, B2, G1 and G2 by TLC. It also gives the procedure for total viable count for bacteria and fungi, qualitative and quantitative determination of *Enterobacteriaceae* and certain other Gram-negative bacteria, qualitative tests for determination of specific organisms such as *Pseudomonas aeruginosa, Staphylococcus aureus* and *Salmonella* species.

The Indian Herbal Pharmacopoeia (2002) recommends the WHO limits for microbial contamination. Very few published reports are available on nature and content of microbial load in Indian medicinal plants. We need to generate our own guidelines for limits and indicator organisms, particularly if botantical medicines are to be sort in the international market.

Microbial contamination of botanicals is influenced by environmental factors such as temperature, humidity, extent of rainfall during the pre-harvesting, harvesting, and post-harvesting periods, handling practices and storage conditions of crude and processed medicinal plant materials. This reflects the importance of indicator organisms and framing of limits for microbial contamination based on the existing environmental conditions in the country. Further, the microbial risk inherent to any botanical may vary with regard to the different stages of the production line and processing factors, which largely determine the microbial quality of the final product. The application of hot water extraction (herbal infusion, herbal tea) usually compensates for microbiological contamination, since it can be expected that boiling water markedly reduces the viable counts by several log units and also inactivates possible pathogens. However, those drugs that are subjected to cold-water extraction (herbal maceration), may host a considerable amount of microbes, and the extraction procedure carried out at ambient temperature usually enables microbial multiplication.

In principle, most quality aspects of botanical drugs can be compared with those considered in the area of food microbiology, since spices, herbs, tea, vegetables, cereals may exhibit similar microbiological tendencies. However, unlike foods, botanicals contain specific compounds of particular pharmaceutical and medical relevance with dose-dependent properties, and are not consumed for a nutritive or relishing function. Moreover, the consumers of medicinal plants are people who undergo some form of therapeutic treatment. This means that toxicological factors, higher risk levels, and hazard classes have to be considered.

The occurrence of mycotoxins in foods and feeds is not entirely avoidable; therefore small amounts of these toxins may be in foods and feeds. A food is deemed adulterated if it contains poisonous or deleterious substance, such as mycotoxins, which may render it injurious to health. Mycotoxins can be considered added poisonous or deleterious substances because their presence in human food and/or animal feeds can be avoided in part by good agronomic and manufacturing practices. UDFDA strategies to minimize mycotoxins in the U.S. food supply include establishing guidelines (e.g., action levels, guidance levels), monitoring the food supply through formal compliance programs (domestic and import) and taking regulatory action against products that exceeds action levels, where action levels have been established.

Pesticide Residues

Medicinal plant materials are liable to contain pesticide residues which accumulate from agricultural practices, such as spraying, treatment of soils during cultivation, and administration of fumigants during storage. Although the use of pesticides in the agricultural sector has greatly reduced the presence of insects, fungi, and molds in plants, prolonged or excessive usage of pesticides ultimately intoxicate the entire plant material causing several health hazards. WHO therefore recommends that every country producing medicinal plant materials (naturally grown or cultivated) should have at least one control laboratory capable of performing the determination of pesticide levels in accordance with the procedure specified in Quality Control Methods for Medicinal Plant Materials. The guidelines suggest that intake of pesticide residue from medicinal plant materials should be less than 1% of total intake from all sources, including food and drinking water.

Chromatography (mostly column and gas) has been recommended as the principal method for the determination of pesticide residues. However, these techniques are not universally applicable. In chromatography, the separations may not always be complete, pesticides may decompose or metabolize, and many of the metabolic products may be unknown. As a result of limitations of the analytical techniques and incomplete knowledge of pesticide interaction with the environment, it is not possible to apply an integrated set of methods that will be satisfactory in all situations. WHO therefore suggests that plant materials of unknown history should be tested for groups of compounds rather than individual pesticides and in cases where the pesticide to which the plant material is exposed is known or can be identified by suitable means, an established method for determination of that particular pesticide should be employed. The European pharmacopoeia defines limits for plant drugs with respect to 34 specific pesticides under Part 1, V.4.6 Pesticide Residues (1995) and offers methods of analysis under Part1, VIII.17 Tests for Pesticides (1995). Limits applying to other pesticides not specified in the V.4.6 text, and whose presence is suspected for any reason, are in accordance with European Community Directives 76/895 and 90/642:in UK legislation the latter limits are given in The Pesticides (Maximum residue Levels in Crops, Food and Feeding Stuffs) Regulations 1994 (SI 1994 No. 1985). USP also provides limits for 34 different types of pesticide residues including organochlorides and organophospherus[256].

The appropriate frequency of testing for pesticide residues in plant drugs should be determined on the basis of historical data for particular materials and the level of knowledge on their sources and pesticide treatments (if any)[257].

Heavy Metals

The term 'heavy metals' has traditionally been used to describe those elements that should be restricted in ingested

[256] The United States Pharmacopoeia and National Formulary (USP24& NF19), (The United States Pharmacopoeial Convention Inc.) 2000, 1888-1889.

[257] British Herbal Pharmacopoiea, British Herbal Medicine Association) 1996.

materials because of their toxic effects. The term includes not only lead but other metals such as chromium, iron, copper, zinc, nickel, and tungsten, some of which are essential nutrients in trace amounts (e.g. copper, iron, zinc) and some of which have relatively low toxicity (e.g. nickel, chromium). Mercury as a noble metal and the 'metalloid' arsenic are also elements, which should be controlled in foods and medicines because of their toxic natures[258]. The British Pharmacopoeia therefore uses the term 'Potentially toxic elements' rather than 'heavy metals.' Contamination of medicinal plant materials with arsenic and heavy metals can be attributed to many causes including environmental pollution and traces of pesticides.

Many herbal products contain undisclosed heavy metals[259,260,261]. The WHO has proposed the maximum amounts of lead and cadmium based on Allowed Dietary Intake values at 10mg/kg and 0.3mg/kg respectively. The methods for determining the content of arsenic, lead and cadmium have been given in Quality Control Methods for Medicinal Plant Materials. Despite these guidelines, testing for heavy metals and other potentially toxic elements by traditional methods can be problematic. Atomic Absorption Spectrophotometry is a more precise technique, enabling individual elements to be assayed, although the instrumentation is expensive. Considerable technical expertise and experience are required to obtain reproducible results. With regard to medicinal plants, the toxic elements

---

[258] Borkowski B, Contamination of plants by heavy metals Farm Pol 50(15) (1994) 697-710.

[259] Ernst E, Heavy metals in traditional Indian remedies, Eur J Clin Pharmacol 57 (2002) 891-896.

[260] Ko R J, Adulterants in Asian patent medicines, The New Engl J Med 339 (12) (1998) 847.

[261] Au A M, *et. al.*, Screening methods for drugs and heavy metals in Chinese patent medicines Bull Environ Contam Toxicol 65 (2000) 112-119.

which may be present in sufficient quantity to cause concern vary from plant to plant as the physiological uptake of these elements varies. Amounts present also depend on the location, varying according to the quality of the soil or aerial pollution. A general screen on plant materials will give a guide as to what specific elements in which plants may be of concern. There have been sporadic reports of heavy metal toxicity following traditional medicine use, however, in most of the cases such toxicity is the result of incorrect manufacturing process for which traditional systems are held responsible. Such incidences highlight the urgent need to address quality control related issues of herbo-mineral preparations so that botanical medicines can retain their credibility as treatments.

Radioactive Contamination

A certain amount of exposure to ionizing radiation cannot be avoided since there are many sources such as radionuclide occurring naturally in the ground and the atmosphere. Dangerous contamination may be the consequence of a nuclear accident[262]. The amount of exposure to radiation depends on the intake of radionuclides and other variables such as age, metabolic kinetics, and the weight of the individual (also known as the dose conversion factor). Even at maximum observed levels of radioactive contamination with the more dangerous radionuclides, significant risk is associated only with consumption of quantities of over 20 kg of plant material per year so that a risk to health is most unlikely to be encountered given the amount of medicinal plant materials that would need to be ingested. Additionally, the level of contamination might be reduced during the manufacturing process. Therefore, no limits for radioactive contamination are proposed.

---

[262] Chan K, Some aspects of toxic contaminants in herbal medicine, Chemosphere 52 (2003) 1361-1371.

Good Practices and Statutory Guidelines

The principal objective of these practices and guidelines is to define basic criteria for the evaluation of quality, safety and efficacy of herbal medicines and thereby assist national regulatory authorities, scientific organizations and manufacturers to undertake an assessment of the documentation/submissions/dossiers in respect to such products. Assessment of efficacy should cover pharmacological and clinical aspects. Effects of active ingredients and their constituents with therapeutic activity should be described and the indications for the use of the medicines should be specified. The requirements for proof of efficacy should depend on the type of indication. Where traditional use has not been established appropriate clinical evidence should be required.

Current Good Practices

Use of 'good practices' ensures that preclinical and clinical studies of new drugs and vaccines conform to acceptable quality standards. The term Current is often prefixed to indicate the cotemporayness. For disease endemic countries to play a greater role in drug and vaccine development, good practices must be followed for study data to be accepted by regulatory authorities, and for the products to be marketed in the rest of the world. All clinical studies supported by statutory bodies must be carried out according to International Conference on Harmonisation (ICH) / WHO Good Clinical Practice standards, regulatory authorities requirements, and Standard Operating Procedures (SOPs). A document published by Tropical Drug Research division of WHO sets out the objectives of Standard Operating Procedures and defines the Investigators' responsibilities when undertaking a clinical study supported by TDR. It provides instructions for planning, performing, documenting and reporting clinical studies, and also provides a useful glossary of terms[263].

Good Laboratory Practices

Current Good Laboratory Practices (cGLP) are the recognized rules governing the conduct of non-clinical safety studies. They ensure the quality, integrity and reliability of the study data. WHO has published a handbook to help those countries wishing to upgrade their laboratories to GLP status. Based on the Organisation for Economic Cooperation and Development (OECD) principles of GLP, the aim of the handbook is to provide laboratories and trainers in disease-endemic countries with the necessary technical information for implementing GLP programmes[264]. The handbook gives an introduction, history of GLP. It also reviews the need for quality standards in drug research and development, GLP training, and the stepwise introduction of GLP. The OECD principles of GLP and compliance monitoring are also provided.

Good Clinical Practices

Current Good Clinical Practice (cGCP) is an international ethical and scientific quality standard for designing, conducting, recording, and reporting trials that involve the participation of human subjects. Compliance with this standard provides public assurance that the rights, safety, and wellbeing of trial subjects are protected; consistent with the principles that have their origin in the Declaration of Helsinki, and that the clinical trial data are credible. The objective of this ICH GCP guidance is to provide a unified standard for the European Union (EU),

---

[263] Juntra Karbwang and Claire Pattou Standard operating procedures for clinical investigators, 2001, World Health Organization, Geneva.

[264] WHO Handbook: Good laboratory practice, Quality practices for regulated non-clinical research and development, 2001, World Health Organization, Geneva.

Japan, and the United States to facilitate the mutual acceptance of clinical data by the regulatory authorities in these jurisdictions. The guidance was developed with consideration of the current Good Clinical Practices of the European Union, Japan, and the United States, as well as those of Australia, Canada, the Nordic countries, and the World Health Organization (WHO). This guidance should be followed in all clinical trials intended to be for regulatory authorities. The basic principles established in this guidance are also applicable to other clinical investigations that may have an impact on the safety and well being of human subjects[265].

There has been significant increase in number of clinical drug trials (particularly phase 3) conducted in developing countries for infectious diseases such as HIV, malaria, and tuberculosis. Laboratory results provided by medical testing laboratories in the region are critical to ensuring the safety of patients and the generation of good quality data. A number of well accepted GCP and GLP guidelines govern the conduct of clinical trials internationally. However, GCP guidelines remain too vague with respect to sample analysis to ensure practical implementation in these laboratories. In their strictest sense, GLP guidelines refer to the analysis of samples from non-clinical studies. A specific set of minimum standards or requirements for practical implementation of clinical trial requirements in medical testing laboratories in the developing world is urgently required[266].

All biomedical research involving human subjects has to comply with established international guidelines that require ethical and scientific review of the research,

---

[265] Guidance for Industry, E6 Good Clinical Practice: Consolidated Guidance, April 1996, U.S. Department of Health and Human Services, Food and Drug Administration, Center for Drug, Evaluation and Research (CDER), Center for Biologics Evaluation and Research (CBER), ICH.

[266] Stevens W. Qual Assur. 2003 Apr-Jun;10(2):83-9.

alongside informed consent. WHO provides operational guidelines to ethics committees to facilitate, support, and ensure quality of the ethical review of biomedical research., These guidelines define the role and constituents of ethics committee and detail the requirements for submitting an application for review. Such review and details of the decision making process are provided with necessary followup and documentation procedures[267].

ICMR and GCP Guidelines

Good Clinical Practices guidelines have categorized herbal drugs into three types.

The first category involves any known plant drug or extract from Ayurveda, Siddha or Unani literature or used by the physicians of traditional systems. These substances are being clinically evaluated for the same indication, which has mentioned in the traditional texts. Second category is of any extract/compound isolated from plant to be evaluated for a therapeutic effect that has not been described in texts or where the method of preparation is different. These should be considered as a new chemical entities (NCEs) and acute, sub acute and chronic toxicity data should be generated before clinical evaluation. Third category includes any new extract/compound isolated from botanical, which has never been used before and has no mention in traditional literature. This also is treated as new drug and should undergo all regulatory requirements before initiating clinical evaluation. Drugs expected to be used in allopathic setting need to undergo all the procedures mentioned for new drugs. These guidelines are not applicable to the drugs, which are used in an Ayurvedic, Siddha or Unani systems.

❒❒❒

[267] Operational guidelines for ethics committees that review biomedical research, 2000, World Health Organization, Geneva.

8 Herbal Pharmaceutics
Stability and Pharmacokinetics

Typically herbal pharmaceutics may include any medicinal or functional food preparations such as phytopharmaceuticals, single or poly herbal formulations, and nutraceuticals made out of botanical materials. This includes two broad categories. First, there are many evidence based formulations and mixures that may or may not be based on traditional knowledge or practices. The second group includes all the traditional or ethnopharmacological preparations. Bringing herbal medications from either group to the market will require a pharmaceutics approach balanced with an understanding of the original context in which the treatment was used.

As an example, Ayurvedic medicines have been used safely for many years on a wide variety of patients. Medications that have not been altered from their original form have de facto gone through a type of safety testing. When a traditional medicine is prepared differently, then it is essential to validate the drug safety to be sure that the effects of the new procedure don't cause harmful effects. In this same way, the value of animal testing to establish safety and toxicity is not as critical if the botanicals are used in traditional forms. Suitable animal models help in understanding the mechanism of action or pharmacodynamics of medicines. However, it is well known that no good animal models exist for many human diseases, such as asthma, diabetes, and rheumatism. The use of modern technology in making traditional preparations more contemporary and scientific is important but it should not compromise the original basis and principles described in tracditional medicine. The following examples highlight some of the concerns of this approach.

Crude Vs Pure Extracts

There has been a long debate about use of botanical materials that are complex and difficult to define chemically. In the past, the reductionist approach has been popular where such materials are only seen as sources of natural product new drug discovery. Many times, such efforts to distill out a single active agent responsible for the drug's effects fail because of loss of natural molecular diversity in crude extract. For instance, *Semecarpus anacardium* is widely used in Ayurvedic medicine for a variety of disorders. Crude extracts were believed to have anti-tumor activities, which were confirmed in animal models of sarcoma and adenomas that showed a statistically significant increase in the life span of the treatment groups. Attempts were made extensively at the National Chemical Laboratory, Institute of Science, Cancer Research Institute and Haffkine Institute under the program of Department of Science and Technology to isolate the active principle by using preparative HPLC coupled with anticancer activity testing of pure fractions. Analysis of its seed oil reveled presence of long chain catechols, however none of these impure forms were active. The entire effort was carried out for nearly four years but could not identify any anticancer compound in pure form. This example and many such others support the Ayurvedic concept of botanical use. The possible explanation for this could be synergism and role of many ingredients together in form of a cluster for desired therapeutic effects. The inability to isolate pure anticancer compound from Semecarpus does not mean it has no therapeutic relevance. The typical strategies of drug research including activity directed fractionation do not necessarily work in case of Ayurvedic botanicals[268]. One possible rationale for the effectiveness of total natural botanicals can be drawn from the basics of Drug-Receptor theory where a typical conformation of drug molecule is required for optimal triggering of a biological reaction. Natural botanicals would have a whole range of intermediate compounds synthesized de-novo during the biosynthesis of variety of secondary metabolites. In this process we expect to get many closely related derivatives of which the best possible conformation triggers the biological response required for therapeutic activity[269]. While these possible explanations are being researched, it is worth asking whether these medicines can be used for their therapeutic benefit even if their mode of action isn't entirely understood.

Drug and Vehicle

Ayurvedic databases give information about how to consume a particular drug either to enhance potency or to reduce toxicity. This advice is called Anupana and means use of vehicles like honey, milk, warm water and such. For example, Semecarpus anacardium, which is used to treat a variety of illnesses but is considered potentially toxic according to traditional advice, needs to be consumed along with butter oil or other suitable fat. It is known in Ayurveda

[268] Pharmacological investigations on Semecarpus anacardium.. Patwardhan B. Ph.D. Thesis, University of Pune, 1995.

[269] Looking for new drugs: what criteria? Sevenet J. J. Ethnopharmacol 1991 Apr; 32(1-3):83-90.

that any wrong use or administration of this plant may give rise to variety of unwanted effects, and some times very serious hypersensitivity reactions. The processing and use of fatty substances is advocated to avoide such toxic effects. The following observations come from an interesting study on experimental animals. In an acute and sub-acute toxicity studies fractions emulsified using tween80 saline produced pronounced toxicity and 100% mortality at a dose of 25mg/kg dose while at this dose there was no mortality in a group that received fractions with peanut oil where there were signs of anabolic effect. In Ayurvedic texts, this plant is considered to have anabolic activities, which could have been undermined in case of a routine emulsion approach[270].

Drug Processing

The Ayurvedic system uses the same botanical material to treat different conditions and to get different activities. The outcome of the treatment depends on the kind of processing that is recommended, such as heating, boiling, or cooling. One example of this can be drawn from a case of *Adhatoda vasaka* or Vasa which is a popular ingredient of Ayurvedic cough syrups. In an attempt to identify its active principle, various solvent extracts were prepared by the cold percolation method. These extracts were tested for bronchodialator activity in suitable animal models. To the surprise of investigators, these extracts showed bronchoconstrictor effects. Scientists could not understand how a potential bronchoconstrictor botanical could effectively work as a cough syrup. Ayurvedic literature threw light on this mystery, stating that Ayurveda Vasa syrup, or decoction, can only be used for treatment of cough while the fresh juice can be used to stop bleeding by applying

[270] Toxicity of Semecarpus anacardium extracts. Patwardhan B. , Ancient Science of Life, 1988, 8 (2), 106.

it on an open wound. When scientists further studied the effects of decoction, they found that it did indeed have strong bronchodialator activity. The entire chemistry of Vasicine and Vasicinone is based on the fact that the alkaloid gets oxidized during a process of decoction and becomes a bronchodialator, while the cold juice can be used to stop bleeding since it also has vasoconstrictor activity[271]. There are many such examples to show that Ayurvedic medicines have a systematic and scientific approach of processing botanical materials that affects their therapeutic outcome. Failing to comply with the complete Ayurvedic processes and adopting short cuts can result into either compromised therapeutic gains or even dangerous poisonous side effects. In such cases it is important to separate whether the preparation of the medicine is at fault or the treatment itself, as has been seen in the cases of metal or mineral Ayurvedic preparations[272].

Dosage Forms

Ayurvedic pharmacy is quite systematically developed. Ayurvedic pills, decoctions, tinctures, wines, teas, linctus, syrups, creams, lotions are described for the method of preparation, use and indications. In a small experiment to find out physico-chemical characteristics of Ayurvedic pills, it was noted that range of such pills respond selectively and differently to parameters like dissolution and disintegration time. The results could classify Ayurvedic pills into three distinct types resembling to routine, enteric-coated and slow-release type of dosage forms[273].

---

[271] Chemistry of Adhatoda vasaka A Monograph,. Atal CK, CSIR Publication, RRL Jammu.

[272] Lead poisoning associated with the use of Ayurvedaaaic metal-mineral tonics. D, Pizent A, Jurasovi Pongra. J. Toxicol Clin Toxicol 1996 34:4 417-23.

[273] Standardisation of Ayurvedic tablets, Patwardhan *et al*, Ancient Science of Life, 1990, Vol 10, 36-39.

Single and Multi-Ingredient Formulations

Ayurvedic databases give information about botanicals that can be used best as single drugs in natural form or in processed form. It also gives a wide range of multi-ingredient combinations, from simple mixtures to complex processed dosage forms. Typically, modern medicine prefers the use of pure materials because they have the advantage of known pharmacokinetics and dynamics as well as more precise dose-response relationships. Still, the use of multi-drug therapy is also gaining recognition in modern medicine particularly in the treatment of diseases like Tuberculosis and AIDS. Ayurvedic multi-ingredient formulations also give such distinct advantages particularly in the area of difficult-to-treat chronic diseases. Diseases such as diabetes, asthma, hypertension, cancer and arthritis have varied etiologies and therapeutic management is required at different levels and at different sites. In such situations, the multi-ingredient approach of Ayurvedic medicines becomes all the more important. Ayurvedic formulary gives thousands of such multi-ingredient preparations and an excellent rationale can be found in the Ayurvedic classics. One such attempt to design a multi-ingredient formulation (Artrex) for the treatment of rheumatoid and osteo-arthritis has been successfully made and the formulation has been tested in a randomized, double blind, placebo-controlled clinical trial. This formulation gives therapeutic benefits to acute conditions of pain and inflammation and it also addresses immunopathological interventions required for long-term management of slow progressive degenerative disease like RA. It has ingredients that have analgesic and antiinflammatory activities similar to NASAIDs and it also has ingredients with immunomodulatory, anabolic, disease modifying and free radical scavenging activities. Thus the formulation as a whole acts as a combination of NSAIDs and DMARDs[274].

Standardization

Addressing standardization in herbal pharmaceutics is vital. For many reasons, standardization needs broader consideration than it has been given in the past. The time when Ayurvedic medicine was developed was technologically very different and therefore the concept of standardization was quite different. During the past thousands of years, the dynamic process of evolution could have affected the identity of natural materials that are described in Ayurvedic texts, altering their medicinal effects. In the process of commercialization, correct identification and supply of raw material to avoid adulteration has become a challenge. In addition, some of the botanical species might have become extinct. Finally, the properties of botanicals as recorded in classics may have undergone change due to time and environmental factors. Considering these and other possiblities, the standardization of Ayurvedic botanicals and medicines is required. However, it may not work to simply apply the typical modern pharmaceutical pharmacopoeial standards to botanicals and Ayurvedic medicines. The concept of active markers in the process of standardization needs a flexible approach in light of the very complex nature of these materials. Many times it is very difficult to identify bioactive markers. In such situations use of group of known chemical markers is advisable.

---

[274] Efficacy of Ayurvedic formulation in Rheumatoid arthritis and Osteoarthritis. Kulkarni, Patwardhan *et. al.*, Ind. J. Pharmacology, 1992, 24, 98; J. Ethnopharmacology, 1992, 24, 98-101; American College of Rheumatology Scientific Meetings, Chopra A., Patwardhan *et. al.*, Florida 1996, Asia Pacific League Against Rheumatism, Singapore 1997.

Towards Novel Models of Standardization[275]

Recently, many international authorities and agencies including the World Health Orga nization, European Agency for the Evaluation of Medicinal Products and European Scientific Cooperation of Phytomedicine, US Agency for Health Care Policy and Research, European Pharmacopoeia Commission, and the Department of Indian System of Medicine have started creating a new mechanism to induce quality control and standardization of botanical medicines. For Ayurvedic medicine and other traditional medicines newer guidelines of standardization are required. A botanical drug or a preparation thereof is now regarded as one active substance in its entirety whether or not the constituents with therapeutic activity are known. This will be a major step in development of new generation standardized botanical medicines. The WHO has published official documents on medicinal plants and WHO Monographs on selected medicinal plants[276]. Global definitions of botanical products are being developed by international cooperations and a new perspective of standardization, validation, safety and efficacy of botanical medicines is evolving, which is a good sign. Multi-component botanical formulations can be standardized with newer techniques such as DNA fingerprinting; High Pressure Thin Layer Chromatography, Liquid chromatography as well as routine pharmacognostic techniques can be employed. Since there are no ready monographs, in-house monographs need to be evolved and critically followed. For example a multi-component botanical formulation (Artrex) designed for the treatment of arthritis contains four botanicals and all ingredients, their respective extracts and the formulation are standardized

---

[275] EMEA ad hoc working group on herbal medicinal products. Keller K, The European Phytojournal, 1998.

[276] WHO Monographs on selected medicinal plants Volume I and II, 1996, 97.

using HPLC and HPTLC fingerprint profiles of markers. This formulation has been granted a US Patent[277]. A new model of standardization should take into account the complex nature of botanical treatments when considering how to evaluate their efficacy and safety.

Clinical Validation

Human beings have used traditional medicines for number of years and as such, their clinical existence can be presumed. However, to bring more objectivity and to confirm traditional claims, systematic clinical trials are necessary. In Ayurvedic medicine research, clinical experiences, observations or available data are the best starting point as opposed to conventional drug research where it comes last. In this sense, drug discovery based on Ayurveda follows a 'Reverse pharmacology' path. While designing a clinical trial on Ayurvedic medicine one has to specify a research purpose. If the purpose is of discovering a new pharmaceutical, then one can select appropriate models of randomized, single or double blind, prospective, parallel, and continuous or crossover studies. All the necessary clinical and laboratory diagnostic tests need to be included in a study protocol and for all the practical purposes such a study will follow all the crucial requirements of clinical study. If the purpose is to validate the efficacy of traditional Ayurvedic formulations, then the study protocol must take the Ayurvedic basis into consideration.

Manufacturing

The conditions at the time of traditional Ayurvedic pharmacies were different. Today, all the Ayurvedic

[277] A method of treating musculoskeletal disease and a novel composition therefor. Patwardhan B. United States Patent No. 5,494,668, February 1996.

medicine manufacture has to be in accordance with Good Manufacturing Procedures, as required by the US Food, Drug and Cosmetic Act. All the critical pharmacopoeial tests such as dissolution, microbial load, pesticide contamination, heavy metal safety and like must be in accordance with global standards. These issues are more elaborated in a separate chapter with help of information, definitions and examples from US FDA guidance for botanicals.

Stability, Pharmacokinetics and Bioavailability

Stability testing is an integral part of pharmaceutical development process because it evaluates the efficacy of a drug in the form that is to be given to a patient. It is routinely performed on drug substances and drug product. Stability studies are used in development phase of drug discovery and in the following[278]: background information for development of new product and to support the manufacturing and distribution of a pharmaceutical product; to develop suitable packaging information for quality, strength, purity and integrity of product during its shelf life; to submit stability information for regulatory agencies and for the determination of shelf life.

There are variety of mechanisms by which drug product may degrade and may result in a wide range of adverse effects such as: loss of activity, change in concentration of active components, alteration in bioavailability, loss of content uniformity, decline of microbiological status, loss of pharmaceutical elegance, patient acceptability, formation of toxic degradation product, loss of package integrity and reduction of label quality.

[278] Carstensen J.T., Rhodes C.T., 2000. Drug stability principles and practices. Marcel Dekker. 3rd ed., vol.107, pp 501-517.

The International Conference on Harmonization (ICH) of Technical Requirements for Registration of Pharmaceuticals for Human use consists of representative of three pre-eminent pharmaceutical areas of the world, the European Union, the United States of America, and Japan. These guidelines include stability testing of New Drugs and products, Photo stability testing, Stability Testing-New formulations, Analytical Method Development, Definition and Terminology, Methodology, Residual or impurities in new drug substances and dosage forms. Working Party on Herbal Medicinal Products (WPHMP) of The European Agency for the Evalution of Medicinal Products (EMEA) suggests guidelines on specifications which include lists of tests, references to analytical and biological procedures and appropriate acceptance criteria used to assure the quality of an herbal substances, herbal preparation and herbal medicinal product at release and during the shelf life. It emphasizes appropriate fingerprint chromatograms, overall methods of assay and physical and sensory tests[279]. World Health Organization (WHO) guidelines are recommended for four zones based on room temperature and relative humidity[280].

In contrast to chemically defined drugs, most botanicals are poorly characterized in terms of their physical and pharmaceutical properties[281]. This includes variable particle size distribution, low bulk density, poor flow, compression properties and hygroscopicity adversely influence on both

---

[279] EMEA., 1999. Working Party on Herbal Medicinal Products (HMPWP), Stability testing of HD, HDP, and HMP, guidelines 25, p. 48.

[280] General guidelines for methodologies on research and evaluation of traditional medicine. World health organization, Geneva, WHO/ EDM/TRM2000-2001, pp 1-73.

[281] Westerhoff K, Kaunzinger A, Wurglics M, Dressman J, Schubert-Zsilavecz M., 2002. Biorelevant dissolution testing of St John's wort products. J Pharm Pharmacol, 54 (12), 1615-21.

physical and chemical stability of botanicals[282]. The hygroscopic nature of extract powder leads to flowability and compressibility problems. Higher moisture contents can lead to a greater the risk of cohesion and adhesion[283]. The presence of variety of phytochemicals like alkaloids, glycosides, phenolics, terpenoids and steroids makes botanicals chemically complex and poses challenge for analytical method development[284]. Moreover, the presence of enzymes like glycosidases, esterases or oxidases plays important role in the breakdown of plant secondary metabolites. This is of significance in the liquid dosage form[285]. The presence of other concomitant metabolites may influence the overall stability. This has been shown for extracts containing organic acids like malic acid or citric acid, which enhance the stability of phenolic compounds. Stability of a botanical as a whole contributes to the stability of individual phytochemicals, which may show differences in chemical stability[286]. These limitations suggest that botanicals need different study design with respect to limits, testing and duration. In this sense, there is a tradeoff where a complex botanical treatment may provide a therapeutic benefit, but without knowing the active components, other

---

[282] Kopleman, S.H., NguyenPho, A., Zito, W., Muller, F., Augsburger, L.L., 2001. Selected physical & chemical properties of commercial H. perforatum extracts relevant for formulated product quality and performance. AAPS Pharm Sci. 3 (4) article 26.

[283] Connors, A., Amidon, G.L., Stella, J., 1985, Chemical stability of pharmaceuticals: A handbook for pharmacists. 2nd edition, Wiley interscience. 123-26.

[284] Bruneton, J., 2001,Pharmacognosy Phytochemistry of medicinal plants. 2nd edition, Lavoiser publication.

[285] Stefan, G., Chantal, B., 2005. The challenges of chemical stability testing of herbal extracts in finished products using state of the art analytical methologies. Current Pharmaceutical Analysis,1 (2).

[286] Bilia, A.R., Bergonzi, M.C., Morgenni, F., Mazzi, G., Vinceieri, F.F., 2001. Evaluation of chemical stability of St. John's wort commercial extract and some preparations. Int. J. Pharm. 213, 199-208

elements of the product may lead to more rapid degradation of the drug.

Stability Studies on Botanicals

Stability studies that have been conducted on botanical medicines have shed light on the importance of this type of research. Long term thermal stability testing showed a very low (less than 4 months) shelf life of hyperforins and hypericins in *Hypericum perforatum* L. commercial extract and very unstable to light, under forced photo degradation[287]. Degradation of Hyperforins was analysed by LC-MS/MS and NMR in *Hypericum perforatum* L in aqueous acidic solution and functional beverages[288]. Stress degradation studies on guggulsterone using HPTLC show degradation in light and under acidic, basic, oxidation and heat conditions[289]. Also, the accelerated and long-term stability testing of the constituents of artichoke and St. John's wort tinctures constituents has been studied and seems to be related to the water content of the tinctures[290]. The degradation kinetics of Curcumin under various pH conditions and the stability of the Curcumin in physiological matrices show that the decomposition of Curcumin is pH dependant & occurred faster at neutral-basic conditions[291].

---

[287] Bilia, A.R., Bergonzi, M.C., Morgenni, F., Mazzi, G., Vinceieri, F.F., 2001. Evaluation of chemical stability of St. John's wort commercial extract and some preparations. Int. J. Pharm. 213, 199-208.

[288] Orth H.C., Schmidt P.C., 2000. Stability and stabilization of hyperforins. Pharm. Ind. 62(1), 60-63.

[289] Agrawal, H., Kaul, N., Paradkar, A.R., Mahadik, K.R., 2004. HPTLC method for guggulsterone II. Stress degradation studies on guggulsterone. Journal of Pharmaceutical and Biomedical Analysis 26 (1), 23-31.

[290] Bilia, A.R., Bergonzi, M.C., Morgenni, F., Mazzi, G., Vinceieri, F.F., 2002. Analysis and stability of the constituents of artichoke and St. John's wort tinctures by HPLC-DAD and HPLC-MS. Drug Dev Ind Pharm. 28(5), 609-19.

[291] Wang, Y.J., Pan, M.H., Cheng, A.L., Lin, L.I., Ho, Y.S., Hsieh, C.Y., Lin, J.K., 1997. Stability of curcumin in buffer solutions and characterization of its degradation products. J Pharm Biomed Anal. 15 (12), 1867-1876.

The stability of ginsenosides (Rb1, Rb2, and Rg1) in aqueous solutions of varying pH studied kinetically at 37^{0}C and degradation were found to be proton- catalyzed reaction[292]. Dehydrative degradation of (6)-, (8)-, and (10)- Gingerol to (6)-, 8)-, and (10)- Shogaol studied by HPLC[293]. Very few studies on stability testing of botanicals in accordance to international guidelines have been reported so far. The variability in these outcomes shows how important it is for each botanical medicine to undergo stability testing in order to be sure that the consumer is getting a viable treatment.

Role of Fingerprinting and Marker Compound

Chromatographic fingerprinting has been in use for a long time for single chemical entity drug substances. The focus of fingerprinting in classical pharmaceutical analysis is to detect and estimate impurity profiles, thereby giving indication of the source of drug substance and the chemical method of preparation. With herbal drugs, the herbal drug preparation entirely is supposed to be active so that the stability study of a single therapeutic marker is not sufficient. The stability of other substances in herbal drug and herbal drug preparation should also be demonstrated.e.g. by use of appropriate chromatogram fingerprint. It should also be demonstrated that their proportional content remains constant. In the case of herbal medicinal products containing herbal drugs or herbal drug preparation with known therapeutic constituents, the variation in content should be considered ± 5% during proposed shelf life to the initial assay value. In case of herbal medicinal product

[292] Miyamoto, E., Odashima, S., Kitagawa, I., Tsuji, A., 1984. Stability kinetics of ginsenosides in aqueous solution.J.pharm Sci.73 (3), 409-410.

[293] Natalie, J., L., Peter, P., 1998. Use of fingerprinting and marker compounds for identification and standardization of botanical drugs: Strategies for applying pharmaceutical HPLC analysis to herbal product. Drug information journal. 32, 497-512.

containing herbal drug or herbal drug preparation with unknown therapeutic constituents, the variation in content should be considered ± 10% during proposed shelf life to the initial assay value. In this case, a marker compound that should be specific for the herbal drug, herbal drug preparation could be chosen for stability study. Single or multiple markers can be used ensure the concentration and the ratio of component in the herbal medicinal product during a stability study. Thus Chromatographic fingerprints and multiple markers give information on batch to batch variation, manufacturing control and stability herbal medicinal product.

Herbal Pharmacokinetics

The study of pharmacokinetics deals with the effects of the body physiology metabolism on a drug or nutritional substance. It is the study of the time course of drug absorption, distribution, metabolism, and excretion. It also concerns the relationship of these processes to the intensity and time course of pharmacological (therapeutic and toxicologic) effects of drugs and chemicals. In other words, a pharmacological effect can only be obtained if the drug itself, or an active biotransformation product, reaches and sustains an adequate concentration at the appropriate site of action in the body. Adequate concentration depends upon dosage and fate of the drug, which in turn depends upon absorption, distribution, metabolism, and excretion of the substance. The bioactive constituents of herbal medicines are chemicals, just like synthetic drugs. Therefore, they both obey the same pharmacokinetic rules. This fact holds true, regardless of the complexity of the herbal composition.

Pharmacokinetics is a tool to optimize the design of biological experiments with drugs and chemicals. It has become increasingly important in design and development of new drugs and in assessment of old drugs. There is a variety of data available on the pharmacokinetics of synthetic drugs. This also includes the toxicokinetics and drug-drug interaction studies. In summary, we can say the pharmacokinetics of synthetic drugs or semi-synthetics, with well-defined chemical structure is widely documented. In comparison herbal pharmacokinetics is an emerging field.

Herbalists have long studied the effect of herbal medicines on the body, but have hitherto paid less attention to the effects of the body on herbal medicines. This dichotomy expresses the distinction in classical pharmacology between pharmacodynamic and pharmacokinetics. For a given dose of any herbal medicine, its physiological effect (or that of its constituents) will be governed by the effective tissue concentration of the remedy, which in turn is determined by pharmacokinetic parameters- the absorption, distribution, metabolism and excretion of its various components. Knowledge of herbal pharmacokinetics can provide valuable information to aid practitioners in prescribing herbs safely and effectively. It is likely that the pharmacokinetics of botanicals follows the same biological rules as synthetics, and as such behaves in a similar fashion.

Herbal medicines are usually not directly introduced into the blood stream, but oral or topical routes of administration are preferred. This renders the study of bioavailability of paramount importance for the active constituents in plants. Bioavailability can be defined as the degree of absorption of active substances into the bloodstream after oral doses. Hence, bioavailability is also a factor of the preparation, which is used to deliver the dose of active substance. Conventional drugs intended for oral use are designed to have good bioavailability. In contrast, phytochemicals are of natural origin and may exhibit unusual or poor bioavailability, which may be further compounded by the choice of dosage form.

The study of herbal pharmacokinetics is quite complex. It involves multile parameters and criteria. First, the chemical complexity of plant medicines and their potential interactions between constituents needs to be considered. Second, the variation in bioavailability of different compounds; third, the active components are often not known. Forth, herbal materials may not have predictable pharmacokinetic characteristics as natural compounds may act like prodrugs that are often metabolized. Traditional medicines use decoctions and aqouous extracts involving large polar molecules, which might have poor and unpredictable bioavailability; the analytical methods are complicated due to the complex chemical nature of botanicals. Lastly, herbal bioactivation also is likely to affect the pharmacokinetic parameters. Still, the study of herbal pharmacokinetics tests the limits of what we understand about science. By taking on the task of trying to understand botanical medicines, we are pushing our ability to understand the human body. Hopefully, the outcome of these studies will help scientists from all drug discovery fields to develop a better understanding of pharmacokinetics.

Knowledge of pharmacokinetic processes can help explain and predict the efficacy and toxicity of herbal preparations. Route of administration, formulation, age, genetic and ethnic factors, renal and hepatic disorders, other pathological factors, smoking, dietary and nutritional factors, and drug interactions all affect pharmacokinetics. Botanical and synthetic drugs are equally affected by these factors. Herbs can induce alterations in the pharmacokinetics of synthetic drugs and vice versa.

Bioequivalence

Two medicinal products are bioequivalent if they are pharmaceutically comparable and their bioavailability (rate and extent) after administration in the same molar dose are similar to such a degree that their effects, with respect to both efficacy and safety, are essentially the same[294].

Herbal extracts can be divided into different categories: Extracts containing constituents with known therapeutic activity; Extracts containing constituents with relevant pharmacological constituents (active markers) and Extracts where the constituents being relevant for therapeutic activity are unknown[295]. Pharmacokinetic study design will be different for different categories of extracts. The most crucial parameter in any kinetic study is the bio-analytical method followed for the study. The proposed method should be sensitive enough to detect compounds of interest in biological samples and at the same time should be selective enough to rule out interfering substances.

Therapeutic Equivalence

A medicinal product is therapeutically equivalent with another product if it contains the same active substances or therapeutic moiety and, clinically shows the same effectiveness and safety as that of innovator product. The criteria for therapeutic bioequivalence of different herbal medicinal products are the same as for chemically defined substances.

---

[294] Committee for Proprietary Medicinal Products. Note for Guidance on the investigation of bioavailability and bioequivalence CPMP/EWP/QWP1401/98 Draft.

[295] European Agency for Evaluation of Medicinal Products Working Party on Herbal Medicinal Products. Points to consider on Biopharmaceutical Characterization of Herbal Medicinal Products.EMEA/HMPWP/344/03 Draft.

Extract categories and parameter useful in bioequivalence studies

Extract	Chemical assay	Bioassay
Silybum marianum	HPLC silibinin	-
Aesculus hippocastanum	RIA under special condition	Venous function test
Kava kava	HPLC kava-pyrones	Pharmaco EEG
Ginkgo biloba	HPLC ginkgolides, bilobalides	Pharmaco EEG PAF inhibitory activity
Hypericum perforatum	HPLC hypericin, hyperforin	Reuptake inhibition of neurotransmitters
Crataegi folium	-	Influence on neuro-humoral paramters
Harpagophytum procumbens	Harpagoside	Influence on COX-1, COX-2, lipoxygenase
Salix purpurea	HPLC, salicyclic acid and metabolides	Influence on COX-1, COX-2, lipoxygenase
Vitex agnus castus	-	Influence on gonadotropins, prolactin
Capsicum annuum	HPLC, capsaicin	
Valeriana officinalis	-	Pharmaco EEG

In comparison, pharmaceutical equivalence involves raw material quality, extraction, manufacturing process, and standardization. Biopharmaceutical equivalence involves the same extract or fractions, the same presentation form, the same dose, and *in vitro* qualitative and quantitative conformity. Equivalence in a bioassay with regards to the pharmacological profile means the same profile in cell cultures, isolated receptor systems, enzymes, isolated organs and in the whole animal. To demonstrate therapeutic equivalence there are two strategies. First, where direct evidence comes from a clinical study with primary and secondary end points regarding effectiveness or clinical studies with pharmacodynamic and surrogates as end points. Second include indirect evidence from analytical, pharmacological or *in vitro* studies in cells systems.

❑❑❑

9

Preclinical and Clinical Evaluation

The development of a new drug begins typically in the chemistry laboratory and is followed by a wide range of biological studies *in vitro* (cells/tissues) and *in vivo* (animals), which forecast what the agent would do in humans. The focus of these studies moves from evaluating the safety of a drug for use in humans to looking at its clinical relevance. Pharmacodynamics involves a set of biological studies both *in vitro* and and *in vivo* to get a better understanding of the mechanism of action of a drug. Preclinical studies mainly include safety and toxicity to ensure its safety for use in humans. Typically, preclinical *in vitro, in vivo,* and Phase I testing may not be necessary if preliminary data on safety are available. However, preclinical data or clinical observations are still necessary to justify a rationale for use and safety in initial clinical studies.

Three main screening approaches are generally used in drug development. Simple Screening evaluates substances that have a particular property by one or two tests. There is no need for a series of tests in which the interpretation of results of one test may depend on others. Blind Screening is used for a new plant extract where no adequate pharmacological information is available. Blind screening may give clues for potential activity and worthiness to probe further for pharmacological activities. Programmed screening involves a new plant extract or substance with known pharmacological effects and results in more precise information.

In vitro Studies

As alternative to animal experiments, increased attention is currently being given to techniques involving cells, tissues, and organs *in vitro*. Although, these studies avoid animal ethics issues and have advantages such as precision and speed, they remain indicative and not confirmative. While there are many good *in vitro* assays, their main problem is that the outcome is removed from the biological context, so the question remains of whether the results are applicable in a human or animal model. Some examples of preclinical studies on plant-derived products using tissue culture technique are given in the following Table 1.

Cell Line Studies

Sometimes it is difficult to obtain human tissue or isolating specific types of cells, which presents a major challenge to *in vitro* studies.. Moreover, handling of human tissue is subject to strict biosafety regulations and its cultureing is subject to ethical regulations. Few examples of use of cell lines are given in in following Table 2.

*In vivo*s Animal Studies

Animal studies involve many pieces of equipment for measuring physiological parameters in the experimental animals, be it mouse, rat, hamster, guinea pig, rabbit, cat, dog, or monkey. Results obtained from these studies provide a broad idea of activity. Some examples of animal studies are given in following Table 3.

Table : 1. Preclinical studies on plant-derived products using Plant tissue culture technique

Plant Source	Drug used	Tissue culture	Activity/Effect
Scutellaria barbata (Lamiaceae)	Flavonoids[296]	Human myometrial smooth muscle cell (SMC) s and leiomyomal SMCs.	↓Tumor cell numbers, arrested cell proliferation & also↓ apoptosis
Traditional Korean medicinal herbs formulation KYH-1.	Aq. Extract[297] of herbal	Surrogate in vitro assays for HBV (hepatitis B virus) & HCV (hepatitis C virus) measured in tissue culture.	Antiviral potency
PADMA 28, a multi-component herbal mixture formulated.	PADMA 28[298]	Human dermal fibroblasts & Epidermal keratinocytes in monolayer culture. Human skin in Organ culture.	"Skin-repairing" agent.

Table : 2. Studies with cell line

Plant Source	Drug used	Cell line	Activity/Effect
Symplocos chinensis	Triterpenoid Saponins[299] "Symplocos-osides G-K"	Cancer cell lines KB, HCT-8, Bel-7402, BGC-823 and A549	Cytotoxicity
Various herbal medicines	Flavonoids[300]	HeLa cell lines	Anti-HP activity
Kadsura anaosma.	Triterpenoid acids[301]	CCRF-CEM leukemia cells and HeLa cells.	Cytotoxicity
Curcuma zedoaria Roscoe & Poncirus trifoliata Raf	Crude extracts[302]	Vero cells	Hypocholester-olemic agents

[296] Kim DI, Lee TK, Lim IS, Kim H, Lee YC, Kim CH; 2005; Regulation of IGF-I production and proliferation of human leiomyomal smooth muscle cells by Scutellaria barbata D. Don in vitro: isolation of flavonoids of apigenin & luteolin as acting compounds; Toxicol Appl Pharmacol.; Jun 15;205(3):213-24.

[297] Jacob JR, Korba BE, You JE, Tennant BC, Kim YH; 2004; Korean medicinal plant extracts exhibit antiviral potency against viral hepatitis; J Altern Complement Med.; Dec; 10(6): 1019-26.

[298] Aslam MN, Fligiel H, Lateef H, Fisher GJ, Ginsburg I, Varani J; 2005; PADMA 28: a multi-component herbal preparation with retinoid-like dermal activity but without epidermal effects; J Invest Dermatol.; Mar; 124(3): 524-9.

[299] Fu GM, Wang YH, Gao S, Tang MJ, Yu SS;(2005); Five New Cytotoxic Triterpenoid Saponins from the Roots of Symplocos chinensis; Planta Med; Jul; 71(7): 666-672.

[300] Shin JE, Kim JM, Bae EA, Hyun YJ, Kim DH.(2005) "In vitro inhibitory effect of flavonoids on growth, infection and vacuolation of Helicobacter pylori" Planta Med. Mar;71(3):197-201.

Table : 3. Studies on various animal models

Plant	Drug used	Animal model	Activity/Effect
Ganoderma lucidum (Reishi mushroom)	Water-soluble polysaccharide (PS) fractions[303]	Rats	Anti-ulcer
Asparagus racemosus	Aqueous extract[304]	Swiss albino mice	Immunoadjuvant
Withania somnifera	Aqueous extract[305]	Swiss albino mice	Immunomodulator
Kohki Tea *(Engelhardtia chrysolepis)*	Kohki Tea, a Japanese herbal drink[306]	New Zealand White rabbits.	Anti-ischemic
Peumus boldus	Boldine, an alkaloid[307]	LDLR (-/-) mice	Anti-atherosclerotic
Herbal medicine	Herbal medicine ND-10[308]	Cynomolgus monkeys	Laxative

---

[301] Chen YG, Hai LN, Liao XR, Qin GW, Xie YY, Halaweish F. (2004) "Ananosic acids B and C, two new 18(13—>12)-abeo-lanostane triterpenoids from Kadsura ananosma" J Nat Prod. May; 67(5): 875-7.

[302] Liu JC, Chan P, Hsu FL, Chen YJ, Hsieh MH, Lo MY, Lin JY. (2002), "The in vitro inhibitory effects of crude extracts of traditional Chinese herbs on 3-hydroxy-3-methylglutaryl-coenzyme A reductase on Vero cells" Am J Chin Med. 30(4): 629-36.

[303] Gao Y, Tang W, Gao H, Chan E, Lan J, Zhou S;(2004); "Ganoderma lucidum polysaccharide fractions accelerate healing of acetic acid-induced ulcers in rats"; J Med Food.; Winter; 7(4): 417-21.

[304] Gautam, M., Diwanay S., Gairola, S., Shinde, Y., Patki, P., & Patwardhan, B. (2004). Immunoadjuvant potential of Asparagus racemosus aqueous extract in experimental system.91, 251-5.

[305] Gautam, M., Diwanay S., Gairola, S., Shinde, Y. S., Jadav, S.S., Patwardhan, B.K., (2004) "immune response modulation to DPT vaccine by aqueous extract of Withania somnifera in experimental system" International pharmacology 4, 841-849.

[306] Levin RM, Leggett RE, Whitbeck C, Murakami T, Kambara T, Aikawa K.;(2004); "Oral Kohki Tea and its protective effect against in vitro ischemic damage to the bladder; Neurourol Urodyn.; 23(4): 355-60.

[307] Santanam N, Penumetcha M, Speisky H, Parthasarathy S.;(2004); "A novel alkaloid antioxidant, Boldine and synthetic antioxidant, reduced form of RU486, inhibit the oxidation of LDL in-vitro and atherosclerosis in vivo in LDLR(-/-) mice"; Atherosclerosis.; Apr; 173(2): 203-10.

[308] Tsusumi K, Kishimoto S, Koshitani O, Kohri H.;(2000); "Amitriptyline-induced constipation in cynomolgus monkeys is beneficial for the evaluation of laxative efficacy"; Biol Pharm Bull.; May; 23(5): 657-9.

The notion that all herbal drugs are free from side effects is not correct. Any plant material contains hundreds of constituents and some of them are very toxic, such as cytotoxic agents, digitalis and the pyrrolizidine alkaloids. However, the adverse effects of herbal drugs are comparatively less than in synthetic drugs. Controlled clinical trials are beginning to establish their efficacy as well[309].

In general, two types of unwanted effects are observed for herbal medicines. First, the intrinsic effects of herbal drugs, which are related to predictable toxicity, overdosing or interactions with conventional drugs. Allergic reactions are examples of this. Second, extrinsic type effects that are related to manufacturing, identification, adulteration, contamination, substitution, lack of standardization and good manufacturing practices.

To combat potential toxicity issues, it is necessary to do toxicity studies. Such studies include Acute Oral Toxicity, Acute Dermal Toxicity,Acute Dermal irritation / Corrosion, Acute Eye irritation / Corrosion, Repeated Dose 28-Days Oral Toxicity in Rodents, Repeated Dose 90-Days Oral Toxicity in Rodents, Repeated Dose Dermal Toxicity 21 days, Repeated Dose Dermal Toxicity 28 days. Special toxicology involves areas in which a particular drug accident occurs on a substantial scale. All of these studies involve interaction with genetic material or its expression in cell division.

Mutagenecity or genetotoxicity are important areas of study as some mutations may result in cancers. Definitive carcinogenicity of ethnopharmacological products may not be required prior to clinical studies unless there is serious

---

[309] Calixto, J.B; (2000), "Efficacy, safety, quality control, marketing and regulatory guidelines for herbal medicines (phytotherapeutic agents), Braz J Med biol Res, volume 33(2), 179-189.

reason to be suspicious of the drug. A detailed guidance on these aspects is provided in separate chapter.

Clinical Evaluation

The World Health Organization has developed a set of constructive guidelines for clinical trials of traditional and herbal medicines. As per the WHO guideline, a multidisciplinary team of investigators should prepare protocols. Clinical trials of phytomedicine should follow good clinical practice guidelines and effectively implement positive and negative control parameters, careful documentation procedures, and rigorous statistical design and analyses. A clinical trial can be defined as any systematic study of medicinal products in human subjects whether in patients or non-patient volunteers that seeks to to discover or verify the effects of and/or identify any adverse reaction to investigational products, and/or study their absorption, distribution, metabolism and excretion in order to ascertain the efficacy and safety of the products.

Design of Clinical Trials

A careful literature search is necessary before initiating any clinical study to avoid possible duplication and to get some useful hints on the study models and methodology. A study protocol is an important document and should be prepared as per the ICH or other relavant guidelines and must be approved by the Institutional Review Board or Ethics Committees. Open clinical trials involve administration of a drug or treatment to a target group of patients where both patients and staff being fully aware of the objectives and consequences. The results are collected, analysed and the response is presented. Several extraneous factors may also affect a patient's response to treatment. One such factor is the placebo response. Just because of such factors, an open trial has limitations and is mainly of use as cursor to further research.

Addition of appropriate control groups who may be treated with a drug of known activity (positive control) or placebo can produce valuable clinical results to make a statistical comparison of the experimental drug efficacy. A trial is called single blind normally when patient is not aware of whether he is being treated with drug or iplacebo. It is called double blind when both the patient and the phisician are not aware of the treatment. This design removes personal bias to reasonable extent and gives best results if patient inclusion is systematically randomized. Protocol development is the most critical part of any trial. Protocol is a detailed document that defines all steps, approaches, materials and methods to be undertaken for that specfic trail. Any devision from the approve protocol is not allowed.

Selection of Patients

Patient selection and distribution in various trial groups is mainly based on age, sex, and severity of illness. If patient's illness is not likely to seriously progress over a long period of time then a crossover design can be used. Here, each patient receives both the treatments in sequence and only the order of treatment is randomized. Thus, each patient serves as its own control. This has an advantage of reducing errors but requires much longer study time. Exclusion criteria are also important part of trial design. Few common grounds for exclusion of patients from study are: Age (generally over 65 or under 18 unless defined by protocol), pregnancy or lactation, concurrent treatment for other disease, severely ill patients or failure to give consent to participation.

Monitoring of Clinical Trials

Several factors must be considered in monitoring a clinical trial. Ethical considerations are of paramount importance. A patient must give his informed consent, stating that he understands the course of treatment with the drug/substance. It is unethical to submit a patient to a treatment or investigation purely to further the research interest of the investigator. Patient compliance presents a second issue to monitoring clinical trials. Compliance can be improved by ensuring patient comfort, convenience and confidence level. An detailed instruction sheet in local languges may be helpful. Further, random samples of blood and urine should be taken for analysis to check traces of drug. For the wellbeing of the patient, it is important to monitor for the safety of the treatment. If a new drug is to be studied, great care must be taken to monitor any possible side effects. Clinical chemistry and hematological parameters should be measured before starting the trial to provide a baseline for comparison. In case of drug related abnormalities, the clinical trial will have to be discontinued.

Documentation is another important issue, and as such the format of recording of results and information should be carefully designed before the trial. A good trial should include Patient's Case Record Forms (CRF) which detail patient name and individual identification, patient's informed consent, age, sex, occupation, history of illness, family history and previous treatments, dosage schedule, recording reason for withdrawal, rating scale or recording sheet and a side effect scale for each examination, and all necessary information from first to subsequent visits. Once a trial is complete, it is necessary to use appropriate statistical tools to analyze the results. If the drug is statistically superior to placebo or positive control, one can conclude that it is effective.

Clinical trials can be broadly classified. Treatment trials involve tests on new treatments, new combinations of drugs, or new approaches to surgery or radiation therapy. Screening trials normally test the best way to detect presence of certain diseases or health conditions. Prevention trials intend to find better ways to prevent disease in people who have never had the disease or to prevent a disease from resurging. These approaches may include vaccines, minerals, vitamins and/or medicines. Quality of life trials or supportive care trials explore ways to improve comfort and the quality of life for individuals with a chronic illness.

Phases of Clinical Trials

There are four phases of clinical trials based on the objectives and size of the study. Typically, a drug must past through all the four phases before it is finally approved.

Phase 1

The objective of phase 1 trials is to determine the maximum tolerated dose in humans; pharmacodynamic effects, the nature and intensity of any adverse reactions, and the pharmacokinetic behaviour of the drug. These studies are often carried out in healthy adult volunteers using clinical, physiological and biochemical observations. At least 2 subjects should be used on each dose. Investigators trained in clinical pharmacology who have the necessary facilities to closely observe and monitor the subjects usually carry out phase 1 trials. Phase 1 trials may be carried out at one or two centres.

Phase 2

These are exploratory trials where limited number of patients are studied carefully to determine possible therapeutic uses, the most effective dose range and to get a more in depth evaluation of safety and pharmacokinetics. Normally, a limited number of patients are studied at different dose levels. These studies may be limited to one or few centres and should be carried out by clinicians specializing in the concerned therapeutic areas who have adequate training and facilities to perform the necessary investigations for efficacy and safety.

Phase 3

The expanded or Phase 3 trials aim to obtain sufficient evidence about the efficacy and safety of the drug in larger number of patients, generally in comparison with a standard drug and/or a placebo as appropriate. Clinicians in the concerned therapeutic areas who have facilities appropriate to the protocol may carry out these trials. If the drug is already approved/marketed in other countries, phase 3 data should generally be obtained on large number of patients distributed over multiple centres primarily to confirm the efficacy and safety of the drug as recommended in the product monograph for the claims made. Data on Adverse Drug Reactions (ADRs) observed during clinical use of the drug should be reported in the prescribed format. The selection of clinicians for such monitoring and supply of drug to them will need approval of the licensing authority.

Phase 4

These studies are performed after the marketing of the pharmaceutical product. Trials in phase 4 are carried out on the basis of the product characteristics on which the marketing authorization was granted and are normally in the form of post marketing surveillance, assessment of therapeutic value, evaluation of treatment strategies used and monitoring of the safety profile. Phase 4 studies should use the same scientific and ethical standards as applied in pre marketing studies. After a product has been placed in the market, a large number of patients may use it and thus any of the effects or unwanted effects that may have escaped due to smaller number during earlier phases may be visible.

Phases of clinical trials

	Phase	No. of patient	Length	Principle purpose
Human Clinical Pharmacology	1	20-100	Several months to 1 year	Evaluate safety, safe dose range and identify side effects.
Exploratory clinical trials	2	Upto several hundreds	Seven months to year	Evaluate effectiveness, further safety evaluation
Confirmatory clinical trials	3	Several hundred to several thousand	1-4 years	Confirm effectiveness, monitor side effects
Post marketing surveillance	4	Varies	Varies	Post marketing evaluation of long term effectiveness, side effects, cost effectiveness

Efficacy and Clinical Studies

Thre is an increased need to evaluate herbal medicines using well-controlled clinical studies to provide necessary scientific evidence base. Those drugs without a long history of use or which have not been previously researched should follow WHO's Research guidelines for evaluating the safety and efficacy of herbal medicines. For herbal medicines with a well-documented history of traditional use, the following procedures for conducting research and evaluating safety and efficacy may be followed. Literature review → Safety considerations → Efficacy considerations → Clinical trials[310]. Testing for efficacy of the traditional and new herbal products in experimental screening method is essential to find the active component and appropriate extract of the plant. On the other hand, there should be sufficient data from *in vivo* and *in vitro*

[310] World Health Organization. General guidelines for Methodologies on Research and Evaluation of Traditional Medicine. Geneva, World Health Organization, 2000.

studies to validate the therapeutic potential claimed. There is a need to establish the pharmacological activities for identifying and comparing the various preparations for potency[311]. Preliminary assessments of efficacy can be obtained through the results of *in vitro* testing and experiments on animals.

Evidence Base and TM/CAM

Modern medicine is mostly governed by demands for evidence-based practice and biomedical research increasingly moves towards molecular approaches in the search for new treatments. However, the public preferences are moving in a different direction where science is not the starting point for decision-making. Concern over side effects of synthetic drugs and a need for more humanistic management of illness have led many people in industrialized countries to consider the use of TM/CAM. There is an economic face to this trend. Americans and Australians typically pay out of pocket for CAM services. Because health insurance policies traditionally have not covered CAM, Americans spend more out of pocket on CAM than on all US hospitalizations. Australians spend more on CAM than on all prescription drugs. Some major American medical insurers are now beginning to cover complementary medical services—a trend which is emerging in Britain as well. At the same time, the majority of people in most developing countries use traditional medicine for their everyday health needs. The economic reality here is that even in the best situations, the medical systems that serve the majority of the population get less than 1% of the national health budget. Thus, through

[311] Chakravarty, B.K. (1993), "Herbal medicines. Safety and Efficacy Guidelines" Regulatory Affairs J; 4: 699-701.

marginalization and policy neglect, traditional medicine research, quality of care and training suffers adversely[312].

Traditional medicine use in many developing countries is on the increase due to limited availability and accessibility of pharmaceutical drugs that are expensive and often unaffordable. Further, there has been rise in antibiotic resistant strains of bacteria and increasing resistance of the malaria parasite to conventional treatments. On the other hand, traditional health care is familiar, available at the local level and is affordable. Therefore, there is no reason to expect that it won't continue to play an important role in healthcare globally.

The need for evidence-based research has been emphasized by the Commonwealth Health Ministers, which reflects the wider climate of determining best treatment through a formal approach to gathering and synthesizing research data. Evidence-based medicine (EBM) has become a worldwide movement in clinical medicine. Such high standards are now being called for by established medicine in evaluating the claims of traditional or complementary health practitioners. Possibly, due to the historical marginalization of TM/CAM, very limited research funding has been allocated to evaluating their claims under an EBM framework. The relatively limited availability of randomized controlled trial (RCT) data has thus led to charges of there being no evidence in support of the effectiveness of TM/CAM. However, "absence of evidence is not evidence of absence" and there is still debate over what constitutes evidence in TM. For example, how does a scientist measure changes in *qi* – a concept of central importance in traditional Chinese medicine or a concept of *Prakriti* – a way to determine individual constitution as per Ayurvedic

[312] Bodeker G, Complementary Medicine and Evidence, Editorial, Annals Academy of Medicine,January 2000, 29 (1).

system? Should the conventional standards of evidence related to modern medicine be applied to the entirely different theoretical assumptions of traditional health systems and therapies? Such research areas of basic principles have remained ignored so far and instead the focus has been on exploiting TM for drug discovery. In order for true collaboration to happen between these medical traditions, researchers must learn about the assumptions of each other's disciplines. There are few interesting studies that indicate a proof of concept. An advanced analytical tool (Herboprint®) based on three dimensional high pressure liquid chromatography has been developed that correlates the Ayurvedic concepts and helps in primary bioprospecting and quality control by giving additional activity support information[313]. Another interesting study has recently reported genetic correlations between the various classifications of human beings based on Ayurvedic concept of Prakriti underlines importance of scientific research in these areas[314,315].

In order to address areas not readily studied using RCT methodology, and also to correctly design and interpret RCTs, observational studies are receiving new attention. Observational studies are based on quantitative epidemiological methods and quantitative sociological methods in which data are collected through observation. In traditional medicine, it may be assumed that a natural experiment is already taking place, in that practitioners are prescribing drugs and patients are using them. Observational research of existing practice allows for a first

[313] Vijay Kumar, US Patent (pending) 2004, Indian Institute of Chemical Technology CSIR, Hyderabad, India.

[314] Joshi K *et. al.*, Genotype-Phenotype correlations based on Ayurvedic concepts. Cold Spring Harbor Symposium on Pharmacogenomics, November 2004.

[315] Patwardhan B. *et. al.*, Classification of human population based on Ayurvedic concept of Prakriti J Alt Complement Med., 2005.

line of data to be collected without the ethical difficulties of assigning subjects to novel treatments. Data are gathered on what is actually happening and what the outcomes are from these interventions. As suggested by Arthur Margolin of Yale University, the validity and ultimate value of RCTs of complementary therapies would be diminished if they were conducted without preliminary foundational studies[316]. Foundational studies should investigate such issues as the reputed efficacy of the active treatment or the reputed non-efficacy of the control treatments.

❐❐❐

[316] Margolin A., J Altern Complement Med 1999; 5:103-4.

10 Regulatory Guidance to Industry[317]

This guidance explains when a botanical drug may be marketed under an over-the-counter (OTC) drug monograph and when FDA approval of a new drug application (NDA) is needed. In addition, this document provides guidance to sponsors on submitting investigational new drug applications (INDs) for botanical drug products, including those botanical products (or *botanicals*) currently lawfully marketed as foods and dietary supplements in the United States. This guidance also discusses several areas in which, because of the unique nature of botanicals, FDA finds it appropriate to apply regulatory policies that differ from those applied to synthetic, semisynthetic, or otherwise highly purified or chemically modified drugs (including antibiotics). In particular, the guidance states that applicants may submit reduced documentation of preclinical safety and of chemistry, manufacturing, and controls (CMC) to support an IND for initial clinical studies of botanicals that have been legally marketed in the United States as dietary

[317] The general information, definitions and examples in this chapter are based on Draft Guidance to Industry for botanical drug products, August 2000 U.S. Department of Health and Human Services, Food and Drug Administration, Center for Drug Evaluation and Research (CDER).

supplements or cosmetics without any known safety concerns.

Definitions

These definitions are mainly from regulators point of view and may not be appropriate in other contexts.

Active Constituent: The chemical constituent in a botanical raw material, drug substance, or drug product that is responsible for the intended pharmacological activity or therapeutic effect

Botanical Product; Botanical: A finished, labeled product that contains vegetable matter, which may include plant materials, algae, macroscopic fungi, or combinations of these. Depending in part on its intended use, a botanical product may be a food, drug, medical device, or cosmetic.

Botanical Drug Product; Botanical Drug: A botanical product that is intended for use as a drug; a drug product that is prepared from a botanical drug substance. Botanical drug products are available in a variety of dosage forms, such as solutions (e.g., teas), powders, tablets, capsules, elixirs, and topicals.

Botanical Drug Substance: A drug substance derived from one or more plants, algae, or macroscopic fungi. It is prepared from botanical raw materials by one or more of the following processes: pulverization, decoction, expression, aqueous extraction, ethanolic extraction, or other similar process. It may be available in a variety of physical forms, such as powder, paste, concentrated liquid, juice, gum, syrup, or oil. A botanical drug substance can be made from one or more botanical raw materials. A botanical drug substance does not include a highly purified or chemically modified substance derived from natural sources.

Botanical Ingredient: A component of a botanical drug substance or product that originates from a botanical raw material

Botanical Raw Material: Fresh or processed (e.g., cleaned, frozen, dried, or sliced) part of a single species of plant or a fresh or processed alga or macroscopic fungus

Chromatographic Fingerprint: A chromatographic profile of a botanical raw material or drug substance that is matched qualitatively and quantitatively against that of a reference sample or standard to ensure the identity and quality of a batch and consistency from batch to batch

Cosmetic: An article intended to be rubbed, poured, sprinkled, or sprayed on, introduced into, or otherwise applied to the human body or any part thereof for cleansing, beautifying, promoting attractiveness, or altering the appearance, or an article intended for use as a component of any such article, except that such term does not include soap.

Dietary Supplement: A product (other than tobacco) intended to supplement the diet that bears or contains one or more of the following dietary ingredients: a vitamin; a mineral; an herb or other botanical; an amino acid; a dietary substance for use by man to supplement the diet by increasing the total dietary intake; or a concentrate, metabolite, constituent, extract, or combination of any ingredient described above.

Dosage Form: A pharmaceutical product type, for example, tablet, capsule, solution, or cream, that contains a drug ingredient (substance) generally, but not necessarily, in association with excipients

Drug: Means articles recognized in the official United States Pharmacopeias or official National Formulary and articles intended for use in the diagnosis, cure, mitigation, treatment, or prevention of disease in man or other animals; and articles (other than food) intended to affect the structure or any function of the body of man or other animals; and articles intended for use as a component of any articles specified above.

Drug Substance: An active ingredient that is intended to furnish pharmacological activity or other direct effect in the diagnosis, cure, mitigation, treatment, or prevention of disease or to affect the structure or any function of the human body.

Drug Product: The dosage form in the final immediate packaging intended for marketing

Food: The term *food* means articles used for food or drink, chewing gum, and articles used for components of such articles.

Formulation: A formula that lists the components (or ingredients) and composition of the dosage form. The components and composition of a multi-herb botanical drug substance should be part of the total formulation.

Marker: A chemical constituent of a botanical raw material, drug substance, or drug product that is used for identification and/or quality control purposes, especially when the active constituents are not known or identified.

Multi-Herb (Botanical Drug) Substance or Product: A botanical drug substance or drug product that is derived from more than one botanical raw material, each of which is considered a botanical ingredient. A multi-herb botanical drug substance may be prepared by processing together two or more botanical raw materials, or by combining two or more single-herb botanical drug substances that have been individually processed from their corresponding raw materials. In the latter case, the individual single-herb botanical drug substances may be introduced simultaneously or at different stages during the manufacturing process of the dosage form.

Plant Material: A plant or plant part (e.g., bark, wood, leaves, stems, roots, flowers, fruits, seeds, berries, or parts thereof) as well as exudates

Single-Herb (Botanical Drug) Substance or Product: A botanical drug substance or drug product that is derived from one botanical raw material. Therefore, a single-herb substance or product generally contains only one botanical ingredient.

Botanicals, Foods and Drugs

Botanical products are finished, labeled products that contain vegetable matter as ingredients. The FD&C Act characterizes a product primarily based on its intended use. For a botanical product, the intended use may be as a food (including a dietary supplement), a drug (including a biological drug), a medical device, or a cosmetic as shown by labeling claims, advertising materials, and oral or written statements.

For the purposes of this document, the term *botanicals* include plant materials, algae, macroscopic fungi, and combinations thereof. It does not include fermentation products such as products fermented with yeast, bacteria, and other microscopic organisms, even if previously approved for drug use or accepted for food use in the United States, nor does it include highly purified or chemically modified substances derived from botanical sources, such as paclitaxel, because these substances can readily be fully characterized. This guidance addresses only those botanical products that are regulated by CDER.

Many botanical products are used widely in the United States and are often marketed as dietary supplements. Under the Dietary Supplement Health and Education Act of 1994 (DSHEA). A dietary supplement statement of the type described above may not claim to diagnose, mitigate, treat, cure, or prevent a specific disease or class of diseases. A botanical product is a drug if it is intended for use in diagnosing, mitigating, treating, curing, or preventing disease. Such a drug product must be marketed under an approved NDA unless the product is excluded from the definition of a *new drug*. Certain products that FDA determines are *generally recognized as safe and effective* (GRASE) may be marketed under FDA's OTC drug monograph system. Refer to Flow chart 1 for Regulatory approaches for marketing botanical drugs.

Marketing A Botanical Drug Under OTC

A botanical product that has been marketed in the United States for specific indication/s may be eligible for consideration in the OTC drug monograph system. Currently, there are several botanical drugs, including cascara, psyllium, and senna, that are included in the OTC drug review. A request to amend an OTC monograph to include a botanical substance should be submitted by citizen petition. There should be publicly available quality standards for such a botanical substance in the *United States Pharmacopeia* (USP). In the absence of a USP monograph, the petitioner should propose suitable quality standards for inclusion in the OTC monograph and simultaneously propose adoption of those standards in the USP. An OTC drug monograph does not ordinarily contain CMC information, however, tests and specifications for a botanical drug product, including its corresponding botanical raw materials and botanical drug substances, need be made part of the OTC monograph. In addition, FDA regulations on current good manufacturing practices

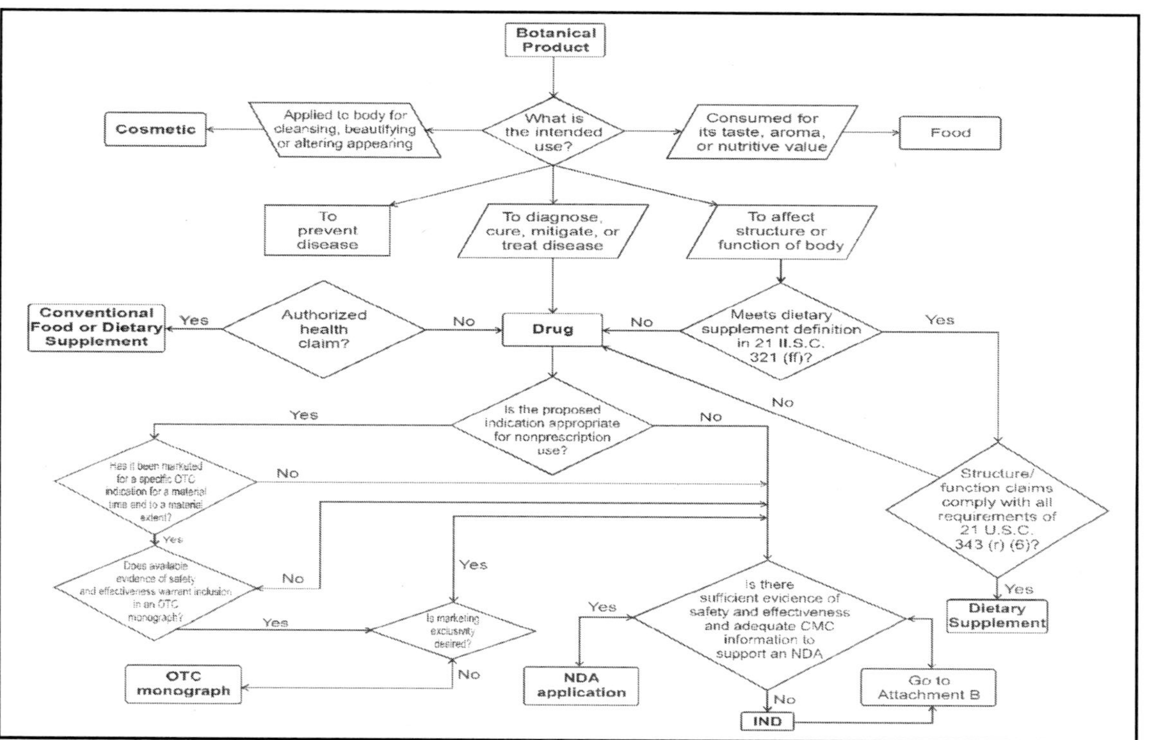

Flow chart 1. Regulatory Approaches to Botanical Drugs. *Source :* US FDA Botanical Drugs Guidance.

(CGMPs) apply to all OTC drug monograph products, including botanical drug products.

Chemistry Manufacuring and Control (CMC) Information

Botanical drugs are derived from vegetable matter and are usually prepared as complex mixtures. Their chemical constituents are not always well defined. In many cases, even the active constituent in a botanical drug is not identified, nor is its biological activity well characterized. Therefore, the CMC documentation that should be provided for botanical drugs will be different from that for synthetic or highly purified drugs, whose active constituents can be more readily chemically identified and quantified. For example, active constituents in a botanical drug might not need to be identified during the IND stage or in an NDA submission if this is shown to be infeasible. In such circumstances, FDA will rely instead on a combination of other tests such as spectroscopic or chromatographic fingerprints, chemical assay of characteristic markers, and biological assay, along with strict quality controls of raw materials and adequate in-process controls and process validation, especially for the drug substance, to ensure the identity, purity, quality, strength, potency, and consistency of the botanical drug.

CMC and Toxicology Information to Support Initial Studies

Many botanical products are legally available in the United States as dietary supplements. Given the wide availability of such products outside of clinical trials, it is important to assess the effectiveness of such products. The preclinical pharmacology and toxicology information that should be provided for legally available botanical products with no known safety issues during initial clinical trials might be much less as compared to synthetic or highly purified new drugs.

INDs for Botanical Drugs

Any botanical drug product that is not generally recognized as safe and effective for its therapeutic claims is considered a *new drug* requires to obtain FDA approval of an NDA or ANDA for that product supported by substantial evidence of effectiveness derived from adequate and well-controlled clinical studies, evidence of safety, and adequate CMC information.

If information available is insufficient to support an NDA for a botanical drug, the sponsor will need to develop further data. If the sponsor wishes to conduct clinical trials in the United States to support an NDA, it will have to submit an IND even if such study is intended solely for research purposes. An IND must contain sufficient information to demonstrate that the drug product is safe for testing in humans and that the clinical protocol is properly designed for its intended objectives.

IND Information for Different Categories of Botanicals

The amount of information to be submitted in an IND for a particular drug product depends on the novelty of the drug, the extent to which it has been studied previously, the drug product's known or suspected risks, and the developmental phase of the drug. For botanicals legally marketed under the DSHEA, there will often be very little new CMC or toxicologic data needed to initiate preliminary clinical (Phase 1 and 2) trials. As long as there are no known safety issues associated with the product and it is used at approximately the same doses as those currently or traditionally used or recommended the IND is allowed. Properly conducted early investigations, including

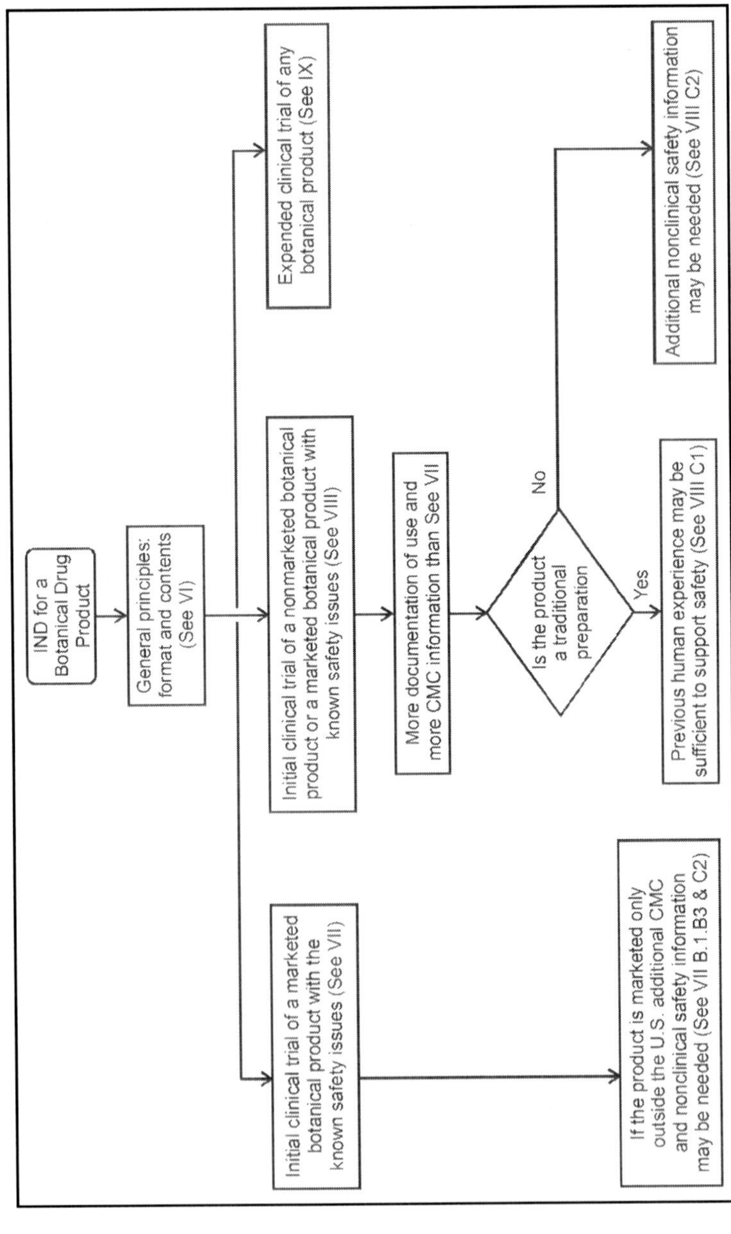

Flow chart 2. Information to be Provided in an IND for a Botanical Drug. *Source* : US FDA Botanical Drugs Guidance.

controlled effectiveness trials in phase 2, indicate if clinical effects are worth pursuing. Botanical drug product showing promise of effectiveness in such early trials may need greater assurance of product quality and consistency and phase 3 clinical studies of safety and effectiveness.

Basic Format for INDs

The format and general requirements for IND submissions include:

1. Cover Sheet
2. Table of Contents
3. Introductory Statement and General Investigational Plan
4. Investigator's Brochure and others as outlined as follows
5. *Protocol:* In general, clinical evaluation of botanical drug products for safety and effectiveness does not differ significantly from evaluation of synthetic or highly purified drugs. For study results to be interpretable, clinical studies should be well designed and carefully executed. A sponsor need not differentiate the clinical effects of each molecular ntity in a botanical product derived from a single part of a plant. Clinical studies of botanical products may pose special problems associated with the incorporation of traditional methodologies, such as selection of doses and addition of new botanical ingredients based on response, which will need to be resolved. In almost all cases, redible studies will be randomized, double-blind, and placebo-controlled (or dose-response). For most conditions potentially treated by botanical drugs (generally mildly symptomatic), active control equivalence designs would not be credible.

For botanical as well as for synthetic or highly purified drugs, absolute safety does not exist for any therapeutic intervention, and any risk should be assessed in light of potential clinical benefits[318]. As with any clinical study, appropriate human research subject rotections must be followed, including submission of the protocol to an institutional review board (IRB) and receipt of proper informed consent. The consent form should describe what is or is not known about the product to be studied and should acknowledge any lack of additional chemical or toxicological characterization.

6. *Chemistry, Manufacturing and Controls:* The requirements for the content and format of the CMC section of an IND require documentation of the drug substance, drug product, placebo, labeling, and an environmental analysis. Plant materials used in the production of botanical drug products often are not completely characterized and defined or are prone to contamination, deterioration, and variation in composition and properties. In many cases, the active constituent in a botanical drug is not identified, nor is its biological activity well characterized. Therefore, unlike synthetic or highly purified drug products, it may be difficult to ensure the quality of a botanical drug by controlling only the corresponding drug substance and drug product. To ensure that a botanical drug product is made consistently with good quality, the sponsor should have, in addition to final product testing, appropriate quality controls for the botanical raw materials and dequate in-process

[318] ICH guidance E1A The Extent of Population Exposure to Assess Clinical Safety: For Drugs Intended for Long-Term Treatment of Non-Life-Threatening Conditions (March 1995).

controls during manufacturing and final process validation, especially for the drug substance.

In the initial stage of clinical studies on a botanical drug, it is generally not necessary to identify the active constituents or other biological markers or to have a chemical identification and assay for a particular constituent or marker. Identification by chromatographic fingerprinting and strength by weight can be acceptable alternatives. Attributes for lot or batch release testing should be determined as the clinical study progresses, although appropriate limits for batch use need not be established until later in phase 3 studies. Batch analyses on clinical lots should be submitted as they become available to demonstrate the batch-to-batch consistency and to help establish appropriate limits for fingerprinting. When possible, efforts should also be made to identify active constituents during phase 3 studies. If a synthetic or highly purified drug or a biotechnology- or other naturally derived drug is added to a botanical drug product, the CMC data for this added substance should be described or cross-referenced according to FDA regulations and guidances. CMC information on a botanical raw material, drug substance, and/or drug product may be submitted by the sponsor as part of the IND or drug master file (DMF).

7. *Pharmacological and Toxicological Information:* The content and format for pharmacological and toxicological information to be provided in an IND are useful in guiding early clinical studies and in predicting the potential toxicity of a new drug. Traditional herbal medicines or currently marketed botanical products, because of their extensive though uncontrolled use in humans, may require less

preclinical information to support initial clinical trials than would be expected for synthetic or highly purified drugs.

8. *Previous Human Experience With the Product:* An IND must contain information about previous human experience with an investigational drug. Because many botanical products have been marketed or tested in clinical studies (although such studies often involve few patients), this information should be included in an IND to assist FDA in its overall assessment of the safety of the product.

INDs for Phase 1 and 2 Clinical Studies of Marketed Botanical Products

This section gives general information for INDs for initial clinical studies on botanical products that have been lawfully marketed and that do not raise safety issues. The ethnopharmacological and traditional medicines along with food or dietary supplements are covered in this category.

A. Description of Product and Documentation of Human Use

1. Description of Botanicals Used

Common or usual names of the plant, alga, or macroscopic fungus; Synonyms (e.g., Latin, Greek, English, Spanish, Chinese); Name of variety, species, genus, and family, including the name of the botanist who first described the species or variety, if known; Chemical class of the active constituent (the chemical constituent that is responsible for the claimed pharmacological activity or therapeutic effect) or characteristic marker (a chemical constituent used for identification and/or quality control purposes), if known;

2. History of Use

History of Use should include information found in historical sources such as books of medical practice in

Ayurveda, traditional Chinese medicine, Unani, Sida and scientific literature about the prior human use of the botanical product, and each of its ingredients, in traditional foods and drugs. The literature should be provided in English (and in its original language, if other than English).

3. Current Marketed Use

Current Marketed Use should include information about the nature and extent of the current worldwide use of the botanical product, and each of its ingredients, in foods and drugs, including evidence concerning its marketing experience in the United States and/or foreign countries. For a foreign-marketed botanical product, the sponsor should provide data (if available) that verify its safe human use, including official proof of the annual sales volume, an estimate of the size of the exposure population, and the rate of adverse effects.

B. Chemistry, Manufacturing, and Controls

Outlined below is the CMC information that should be submitted and Literature references and relevant official compendia or published standards should be provided wherever possible.

1. Botanical Raw Material

The information discussed in section VII.A.1 should be provided for all currently lawfully marketed products. A certificate of authenticity signed by a trained botanist should be provided, if available, for each botanical raw material in a product that is only marketed outside the United States.

2. Botanical Drug Substance

The type of *manufacturing process* (e.g., pulverization, decoction, expression, aqueous extraction, or ethanolic extraction) should be provided, if available. This is especially important where more than one process exists in the literature on which the safety of the botanical drug substance is based.

3. Botanical Drug Product

A botanical drug product is manufactured from a botanical drug substance by adding one or more excipients, mixing, blending, granulating, tableting, encapsulating, or performing other dosage form-specific procedures, followed by packaging. When packaged without further processing, a botanical drug substance is considered the drug product. The following information should be provided for a botanical drug product:

a. A *qualitative description* of the finished product, including the dosage form, route of administration, names of all ingredients (i.e., botanical drug substance and excipients), and a statement that the product is not adulterated with potent, toxic, or addictive botanical substances, synthetic or highly purified drugs, or biotechnology- or other naturally derived drugs.

b. The *composition or quantitative description* of the finished product (i.e., the quantity of the botanical drug substance) expressed in terms of amount per dosage unit. This information should be provided in tabulated form.

Example for a single-herb botanical drug product:

Component	Amount per 1-g tablet
Senna leaf extract (1:8 powdered aqueous extract)	250 mg

Example for a multi-herb botanical drug product:

Component	Amount per 1-g tablet
A 1:5 powdered, aqueous extract from 1:1 mixture of *Forsythia suspensa* Vahl. flowers and *Lonicera japonica* Thunb. Fruits	600 mg

c. If available, the *manufacturer's certificate of analysis* for the study product or *authorization to allow FDA to cross-reference* its previous submission for the relevant CMC information. If this information is unavailable for a foreign-marketed product, the sponsor should perform *quality testing* on the product according to the recommendation listed a heavy metal analysis, and an animal safety test, if applicable, and should provide the *test results* in the IND. The study product should be from a single source and, where feasible, from a single batch. A product sample from the batch to be used in the clinical study should be retained for possible future testing by FDA.

4. Placebo

The components of any placebo used should be described.

5. Labeling

The following labeling information should be provided:

a. A copy of the container label and the immediate outer carton label of the marketed product to be used in the clinical study.

b. A mock or printed representation of the proposed container label that will be provided to the investigators in the proposed clinical study. It should contain the following information: protocol number;

patient number; sponsor's name; product name or code number; strength and/or potency; recommended storage conditions; lot number; statement - Caution: New drug Limited by Federal law to investigational use. In a placebo-controlled clinical trial, both the study drug and the placebo should be properly labeled to protect the integrity of the blinded study.

6. Environmental Assessment or Claim of Categorical Exclusion

A claim for categorical exclusion from the requirement for preparation of an environmental assessment (EA) ordinarily can be made for an IND.

C. Pharmacology/Toxicology Information

1. All Marketed Botanical Products

To support initial clinical trials (phase 1 and phase 2) of a botanical drug product, previous human experience and available animal toxicity data concerning the clinical formulation and the individual botanical ingredients within the formulation should be provided to support the proposed use. As noted in section VI.A, initial studies for U.S.-marketed products may generally be conducted without further pharmacologic/toxicologic testing. Nevertheless, available information should be provided. A database search should be conducted, when feasible, to identify information relevant to the safety and effectiveness of (1) the final formulation of the intended commercial botanical drug product, (2) the individual botanical ingredients, and (3) the known chemical constituents of the botanical ingredients.

An integrated summary of available data from medical and toxicological databases (e.g., Medline, Toxline, TOMES, RTEC) should be submitted for review. Using the information gathered from this literature, the sponsor should address, as appropriate for the proposed study, the following issues concerning the botanical drug product: (1) general toxicity; (2) target organs or systems of toxicity; (3) teratogenic, carcinogenic, or mutagenic potential of any botanical ingredient in the product; (4) relationship of dosage and duration to toxic responses; and (5) pharmacological activity.

2. Foreign-Marketed Botanical Products

For the reasons discussed in section VI, for a botanical product with which there is some foreign marketing experience, but which is not marketed in the United States, in addition to information listed above, the sponsor should provide data that support safe human use and should include the annual sales volume, an estimate of the size of the exposure population, and available data on the rate of adverse effects. The nature of preclinical pharmacology/toxicology information needed before a sponsor conducts an initial clinical study will be determined on a case-by-case basis depending on the indications, dose proposed, and available supporting safe human experience.

D. Bioavailability

Depending on the complexity of the botanical drug product to be studied, pharmacokinetic and pharmacodynamic information may be helpful in the design and interpretation of clinical studies. Botanical products often consist of more than one chemical constituent. In some cases, a products active moieties may not be known, and standard pharmacokinetic measurements to demonstrate systemic exposure to a product in animals and/or humans may be infeasible. However, when feasible a sponsor should attempt to monitor the blood levels of known active ingredients, representative markers, or major chemical constituents in a botanical drug product.

E. Clinical Considerations

The initial clinical trial for a botanical product marketed under the DSHEA should ordinarily be a well-controlled study capable of demonstrating effectiveness. Because the product is marketed and the dose thought to be appropriate and well tolerated is known, there should be little need for pilot or typical phase 1 studies, and uncontrolled observations are unlikely to be useful. Sponsors are therefore strongly encouraged to initiate more definitive trials early in the development program to determine whether a botanical preparation has efficacy for one or more claimed indications. If there is doubt about the best dose of the product tested, a randomized, parallel, dose-response study may be particularly useful as an initial trial.

Regarding the safety of the drug, a botanical preparation lawfully marketed in the United States will be considered acceptable for at least short-term (e.g., up to several months) use in clinical trials. For foreign marketed botanical products, safety considerations will be based on available CMC, pharmacology, and toxicology information, as well as indications, dose proposed, and available data supporting safe human use.

The IND requirements of phase 1 and phase 2 clinical trials for non marketed products are different and more demanding however, they are excluded from this section since the ethopharmacological and traditional medicines are substances already in use and have human consumption history.

INDs for Phase 3 Clinical Studies of All Botanical Products

When conducting expanded (i.e., phase 3) clinical studies on a botanical drug product, an IND sponsor is expected to provide more detailed information on CMC and preclinical safety than when conducting a phase 1 or phase 2 studies. The better definition of the product will ensure an ability to apply data from trials to a well-controlled, reproducible substance. The additional toxicology data is needed to support wider use. This additional information should be provided regardless of whether the product is currently lawfully marketed in the United States or elsewhere as a dietary supplement.

For phase 3 clinical studies of a botanical product, most of the basic information similar to Phase 1 and 2 is needed along with some detailed and more demanding data to ensure quality, safety and efficacy.

A. Description of Product and Documentation of Human Experience

This is similar to earlier sections on how to describe the botanical product and human experience with it.

B. Chemistry, Manufacturing and Controls

To support phase 3 clinical trials using a botanical product, regardless of its marketing experience in the United States or other countries, the following CMC information should be provided unless already submitted in the IND for phase 1/phase 2 studies on the product:

1. Expanded Clinical Studies

A. BOTANICAL RAW MATERIAL

A *description* of the botanical raw material as outlined earlier. If the botanical has no documented history of use, this should be indicated. Proper identification by trained personnel of the plant, plant parts, alga, or macroscopic fungus used, including organoleptic, macroscopic, and microscopic examination, should be provided. If more than one variety or source of a given species is used, they should be blended in a fixed proportion in a consistent manner. A voucher specimen of the plant or plant parts should be retained for every batch. In addition, a certificate of authenticity and information on the grower and/or supplier, growing conditions (including pesticides used), harvest location, harvest time, preservation procedures, handling, and shipping should be provided.

A chromatographic fingerprint of each botanical raw material and the *chemical identity* of the active constituents or characteristic markers in the botanical raw material.

The name and address of the botanical raw material *manufacturer* (processor).

A description of the *preparation* of the botanical raw material, including collection, washing, drying, preservation, and/or detoxification and preservation procedures is needed. Equipment and quantity used, temperature employed, processing time, in-process controls, and yield should be specified.

The *quality control tests* applied by the botanical raw material supplier, including the following specifications: Botanical identification; Chemical identification by spectroscopic or chromatographic fingerprint; Chemical identification for active constituents or characteristic markers if active constituents are not known; Assay for active constituents or characteristic markers if active constituents are not known; Biological assay; Heavy metals; Microbial limits; Residual pesticides, including parent pesticides and their major toxic metabolites; Adventitious toxins (e.g., aflatoxins); Foreign materials and adulterants.

A specimen of the botanical raw material retained as the *reference standard* for use in identification, fingerprinting, and other comparative and noncomparative tests.

A *certificate of analysis* for a representative batch of the botanical raw material.

A description of the *storage conditions*, including the container/closure system and temperature.

B. BOTANICAL DRUG SUBSTANCE

A *qualitative and quantitative description* of the drug substance and the name and address of the *manufacturer* as per given earlier.

A *chemical identification* of the active constituents or characteristic markers in the drug substance is needed. If the chemical identity is unknown, a representative chromatographic fingerprint may suffice.

Appropriate *specifications* (tests, methods, and acceptance criteria) for the botanical raw material, similar to the list of quality control specifications as earlier need to be established by the botanical drug substance manufacturer. Upon receipt of each batch of the raw material and its certificate of analysis, the manufacturer should, at a minimum, conduct an identification test and assay.

A description of the *manufacturing process* for the botanical drug substance should include the quantity of botanical raw material, equipment, solvents, temperature/ time for mixing, grinding, extraction and/or drying, yield, and in-process controls. The yield of the process, expressed as the amount of the extract relative to the amount of the original botanical raw material, should also be indicated. If more than one botanical raw material is introduced to produce a multi-herb substance, the quantity of each raw material and the sequence of addition, mixing, grinding, and/or extraction should be provided. If a multi-herb substance is prepared by combining two or more individually processed botanical drug substances, the process leading to each botanical drug substance should be described separately.

The *quality control tests*, including, but not limited to, the following specifications: Appearance, Chemical identification by spectroscopic or chromatographic fingerprints; Chemical identification for the active constituents or, if unknown, the characteristic markers; Chemical assay for the active constituents, or the characteristic markers if the active constituents cannot be determined. If several botanical raw materials are combined to produce a multi-herb substance and a quantitative determination of each individual active constituent or marker is infeasible, a joint determination can be carried out for several active constituents or markers. Biological assay; Strength by weight; Residue on ignition; Water content; Residual solvents; Heavy metals; Microbial limits; Animal safety test, if applicable; Residual pesticides; Radioisotope contaminants, if applicable; Adventitious toxins (e.g., aflatoxins); Endogenous toxins (e.g., pyrrolizidine alkaloids) and other attributes specific to the botanical raw materials from which the drug substance is derived need to be provided.

A description of all *test methods* and, where appropriate, their validation reports.

A description of the batch of botanical drug substance designated as the *reference standard* for use in fingerprinting and other comparative tests.

Test results for a representative batch (i.e., *batch analysis*).

A description of the *container and closure* used to package the botanical drug substance.

Sufficient *stability data* on the drug substance to support its safe use during clinical studies.

Stability-indicating analytical methods should be established.

Information on the *container label* as described earlier.

C. BOTANICAL DRUG PRODUCT

A *qualitative description and the composition* of the dosage form and the name and address of the *manufacturer*.

Appropriate *acceptance specifications* established by the botanical drug product manufacturer for the botanical drug substance, similar to the quality control tests described earlier. Upon receipt of each batch of the drug substance and its certificate of analysis, the manufacturer should, at a minimum, conduct an identification test and assay.

A description of the *manufacturing process*, without the actual batch record. The description should include weighing, mixing, blending, sieving, in-process controls, and other processes, as appropriate.

The *quality control tests*, including, but not limited to, the following specifications: Appearance, Chemical identification by spectroscopic or chromatographic fingerprints; Chemical identification for the active constituents or, if unknown, the characteristic markers; Chemical assay for active constituents or, if unknown, the characteristic markers; Biological assay; Strength by weight; Residual solvents; Microbial limits; dventitious toxins (e.g., aflatoxins) and other attributes specific to the dosage form of interest.

A description of all *test methods* and, where appropriate, their validation procedures.

Test results for a representative batch

A description of the *container and closure* used to package the finished product

Sufficient *stability data* on the drug product to support its safe use during clinical studies. Stability-indicating analytical methods should be established.

D. PLACEBO AS PER EARLIER

E. LABELING AS PER EARLIER

F. EA OR CLAIM OF CATEGORICAL EXCLUSION

2. End-of-Phase 3 Clinical Studies and Pre-NDA Considerations

By the end of the phase 3 clinical trial, as the sponsor prepares to submit an NDA, the following objectives should be reached:

a. Adequate controls for *botanical raw materials* should be established.

b. The *manufacturing process* should be finalized and validated, and *in-process controls* should be established. An executed batch record should be available.

c. *Batch-to-batch consistency* should be demonstrated for the botanical drug substance and drug product based on results from all chemical, physical, and biological tests on all relevant batches. All chemical constituents present in the drug substance batches should be qualitatively and quantitatively comparable based on spectroscopic and/or chromatographic fingerprinting.

d. Appropriate *specifications* (i.e., a list of test attributes, analytical methods and test procedures, and acceptance criteria), including identification and assay for active constituents, identification and assay for characteristic markers, and/or biological assay, should be established to control the quality of the drug substance and product. Both the active constituents and the biological assay should be clinically relevant. If the identity of the active constituents is not known or a suitable assay cannot be developed, the characteristic markers should be demonstrated to be clinically relevant by direct or indirect correlation to the clinical outcome.

e. *Analytical methods and test procedures* should be properly validated. Analytical methods used for fingerprinting should be capable of detecting as many chemical constituents as possible. Multiple fingerprints, using a combination of analytical methods with different separation principles and test conditions, may be useful. Additionally, the analytical methods in combination should be able to demonstrate the mass balance of the test sample.

f. A suitable *reference standard* for each of the botanical raw materials, drug substances, and drug product should be established and retained.

g. *Stability-indicating analytical methods* should be developed to monitor the stability of the drug substance and drug product. The stability of a botanical drug substance or product generally should not be based entirely on the assay of the active constituents, assay of the characteristic markers, or biological assay, because degradants formed during storage from other chemical constituents in the botanical drug substance or product should also be controlled. An analytical method capable of detecting these degradants (such as a chromatographic fingerprint) should be established through exploratory studies by subjecting the drug substance and drug product to stress conditions.

h. A comparison of the similarities and/or differences in CMC among the preclinical, clinical, and intended commercial products should be made regarding raw materials, drug substance, and drug product.

i. The manufacturing and testing facilities for the drug substance and drug product should be ready for FDA inspection to determine if they are in conformance with CGMPs. A satisfactory inspection is necessary for NDA approval.

Applicants are encouraged to discuss with the review division any CMC issues regarding a botanical drug prior to the preparation and submission of an NDA.

C. Preclinical Safety Assessment (Including Pre-NDA)

To support safety for expanded clinical studies or to support marketing approval of a botanical drug product, toxicity data from standard toxicology studies in animals may be needed. A botanical product submitted for approval for marketing as a drug will be treated like any other new drug under development. Previous human experience may be insufficient to demonstrate the safety of a botanical product, especially when it is indicated for chronic therapy. Systematic toxicological evaluations could be needed to supplement available knowledge on the general toxicity, teratogenicity, mutagenicity, and carcinogenicity of the final botanical product. Depending on the indication (e.g., target patient population, disease to be treated), route of administration, and duration of recommended drug exposure, the timing of these animal studies in relation to concurrent clinical trials and other requirements for preclinical animal studies can vary.

The following are points to consider in preparing a preclinical pharmacology / toxicology development plan for a botanical drug product that is intended to be used in large-scale human trials or to support an NDA. If questions arise during any stage of the clinical development of a botanical drug, sponsors are encouraged to consult the appropriate review division in CDER.

1. Repeat-Dose General Toxicity Studies

The primary objective of long-term, repeat-dose toxicity studies in animals is to identify the target organs and/or systems for toxicity and the threshold doses for producing toxic effects. The studies provide information valuable for designing long-term clinical studies at safe doses with appropriate monitoring for predicted adverse reactions. Existing literature on the animal toxicity of a botanical drug product is often limited to single-dose (acute) toxicity studies. These studies may be inadequate to support the conclusion that a botanical drug product is *nontoxic* for multiple administrations because they were not designed to monitor the usual parameters of toxicity (e.g., clinical pathology and histopathology) or take into consideration the effect of more frequent dosing.

To support expanded clinical trials, repeat-dose toxicity of a drug product should usually be evaluated in two mammalian species (one of which is a non-rodent) by employing sufficiently high doses to produce a toxic effect or by using a maximum feasible dose. If possible, the drug should be tested using the same formulation and route of administration as proposed for clinical use. Animal studies should be of a duration at least equal to that of the clinical trial (usually a minimum of two weeks). General animal toxicity studies need not exceed 6 months of testing in a rodent species and 9 months testing in a non-rodent species[319].

[319] International Conference on Harmonisation (ICH) guidance M3 Nonclinical Safety Studies for the Conduct of Human Clinical Trials for Pharmaceuticals (November 1997).

2. Nonclinical Pharmacokinetic/Toxicokinetic Studies

In the development of a new drug that is a single molecular entity, pharmacokinetic studies are often carried out to demonstrate systemic exposure and to relate exposure levels to toxicities in both animals and humans. Because botanical products usually consist of more than one chemical constituent, standard pharmacokinetic measurements to substantiate the systemic exposure of a botanical drug product in animals may be technically infeasible. However, monitoring major or representative chemical constituents in a botanical drug product can provide valuable information regarding systemic exposure. Depending on the complexity of the botanical drug product to be studied, pharmacokinetics could be helpful in the design and interpretation of toxicity studies[320].

3. Reproductive Toxicology

Reproductive toxicology studies, such as those on fertility/reproductive performance, teratology, and prenatal/perinatal development in animals, provide information on the potential of a botanical drug product to produce toxicity during the different stages of reproductive and developmental processes. In the absence of documentation on reproductive toxicity in humans or animals, these tests should be conducted prior to expanded clinical trials[321].

4. Genotoxicity Studies

Information on the potential of a botanical drug product to produce genetic toxicity should be obtained as early as

---

[320] ICH guidances S3A Toxicokinetics: The Assessment of Systemic Exposure in Toxicity Studies (March 1995), and S3B Pharmacokinetics: Guidance for Repeated Dose Tissue Distribution Studies (March 1995).

[321] The ICH guidances S5A Detection of Toxicity to Reproduction for Medicinal Products (September 1994), and S5B Detection of Toxicity to Reproduction for Medicinal Products: Addendum on Toxicity to Male Fertility (April 1996).

possible, preferably before the initiation of human clinical trials. A complete assessment of genetic toxicity may be needed prior to expanded clinical trials[322]. If the tests chosen indicate that a drug is devoid of genetic toxicity, additional studies may not be needed. If one or more test results are positive, the sponsor may need to carry out additional genotoxicity tests in consultation with the appropriate CDER review division.

5. Carcinogenicity Studies

Carcinogenicity studies may be needed to support marketing approval of a botanical drug, depending on the duration of therapy or any specific cause for concern. The toxicity profile of the botanical drug product and the indication and duration of the intended use may influence the need for carcinogenicity studies and their timing relative to clinical development. Draft protocols for carcinogenicity studies should be submitted to the appropriate review division and the CDER Carcinogenicity Assessment Committee for review and concurrence prior to the initiation of such studies to ensure the acceptability of dose selection and study design. Study types should be in accordance with the ICH guidelines[323].

6. Special Pharmacology/Toxicology Studies

A general evaluation of pharmacological activity on organs and/or systems is often performed during new drug

[322] ICH guidances S2A Specific Aspects of Regulatory Genotoxicity Tests for Pharmaceuticals (April 1996), and S2B Genotoxicity: A Standard Battery for Genotoxicity Testing of Pharmaceuticals (November 1997).

[323] ICH guidance S1A The Need for Long-Term Rodent Carcinogenicity Studies of Pharmaceuticals (March 1996; ICH guidance S1B Testing for Carcinogenicity of Pharmaceuticals (February 1998); ICH guidances S1C Dose Selection for Carcinogenicity Studies of Pharmaceuticals (March 1995), and S1C(R) Dose Selection for Carcinogenicity Studies of Pharmaceuticals: Addendum on a Limit Dose and Related Notes (December 1997).

development. This evaluation can be accomplished using established in vitro and in vivo assays of broad specificity that screen for the modes and sites of action of the botanical drug. When significant and unique toxicities to certain organs and/or systems are evident, the sponsor should provide further explanation of the mechanism of toxic actions, if necessary by performing additional in vitro or in vivo studies.

7. Regulatory Considerations

Preclinical toxicity studies conducted as part of botanical drug development and intended to support safety must be in accordance with regulations governing good laboratory practices. To the extent possible, a botanical drug substance tested in animals should be prepared and processed in the same manner, and the botanical drug product should have the same formulation, as the product intended for human use. Both the drug substance and the drug product should be made with batch-to-batch consistency. If changes occur in the drug substance or product during clinical development, bridging toxicity studies might be needed.

D. Bioavailability and Drug-Drug Interactions

The general requirements for, and criteria for waiver of, *in vivo* bioavailability data in an NDA, are applicable to botanical drug products. These data should be obtained from properly designed *in vivo* bioavailability studies during the IND stage. The type of bioequivalence study that is appropriate for a specific botanical drug product is based on the following: (1) information on the active constituent, if known; (2) the complexity of the drug substance; and (3) the availability of analytical methods. FDA may, for good cause, waive or defer the in vivo bioavailability study requirement if a waiver or deferral is compatible with the protection of the public health.

Because there could be more than one active constituent in a botanical drug product or the active constituent may not be identified, it could be difficult or impossible to perform standard in vivo bioavailability and pharmacokinetics studies by measuring, as a function of time, the concentration of the active moiety, active ingredients, or active metabolites in whole blood, plasma, serum, or other appropriate biological fluid, or by measuring the excretion of the active moiety or active metabolites in urine. In some cases, it may be possible to measure an acute pharmacological effect as a function of time using an appropriate biological assay method. If this is not possible, the bioavailability and pharmacokinetics of a botanical drug could be based on clinical effects observed in well-controlled clinical trials.

Interactions with other commonly used medicines, either synthetic/highly purified or botanical, may occur with botanicals and should be investigated extensively. This may include characterization of the metabolic enzymes and/or pathway affected by the drug.

Where possible, the effects of impaired clearance (renal or hepatic) on the drug's pharmacokinetics should be examined. This is easiest when the active substance(s) are known, but even if they are not, knowledge of the major constituents should make it possible to determine the effects of impaired clearance. Dose-response information may indicate the proper level of concern about impaired excretion.

As with synthetic and/or highly purified drugs, pharmaceutical and biopharmaceutical studies for botanical drug products are important for product quality control, batch comparison, and linkage between different strengths. These studies may involve, for example, in vitro dissolution testing, in situ drug absorption testing, in vitro-in vivo correlation studies, or in vitro percutaneous absorption/ penetration testing, depending on the indication and formulation of the botanical product.

E. Clinical Considerations

Expanded studies of botanicals have the same purposes as expanded studies of synthetic drugs, including further evaluation of dose-response for favorable and unfavorable effects and evaluation of long-term effectiveness, different populations, different stages/severity of disease, and drug-drug interactions.

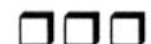

11 Validating Health Claims and Pharmacoepidemiology

Review of Health Claims

Regulators of different countries have different procedures and views to review health claims of traditional medicine, herbal medicines, botanicals, functional foods, nutraceuticals, health products, diatory supplements and such other natural forms of materials intended to use for health promotion. However, if such products carry any therapeutic or health benefit claims then the regulators may provide general guidance and demand for sufficient evidence base in support of such claims. For instance, U. S. Food and Drug Administration, Center for Food Safety and Applied Nutrition (CFSAN) provides general guidance to review of health claims in functional foods and dietary supplements. Ethnopharmacological preparations involving herbal medicine and traditional medicines prepared from natural ingredients also will need similar process. The scientific review process for health claims of such products is comprehensive and mainly focuses on review of individual studies[324].

[324] Food Advisory Committee, Interpretation of Significant Scientific Agreement in the Review of Health Claims, CFSAN, US FDA, Working Group Final Report,1999.

Types of Studies

A health claim review may range from human studies to *in vitro* laboratory investigations. Most clinical and epidemiological studies of humans can be divided into interventional studies and observational studies. In an interventional study, the investigator controls whether the subjects receive an exposure or an intervention whereas in an observational study, the investigator does not have control over the exposure or the intervention. In general, interventional studies provide the strongest evidence for an effect of treatment. Regardless of the inherent strengths and weaknesses of the study design, the overall quality of each individual study is paramount in assessing its contribution to the weight of the evidence for the proposed substance / disease relationship. A well-designed and conducted observational study is more persuasive and should be accorded greater weight than a poorly designed and conducted interventional study.

The "gold standard" of interventional studies is the randomized controlled clinical trial. In a randomized controlled trial, subjects similar to each other are randomly assigned either to receive the intervention or not to receive the intervention. The subjects are not preferentially selected to receive the intervention being studied. The researcher who assesses the outcome also may not know which subjects received the intervention. This removes selection and treatment bias. Such studies are often given the most weight and can provide the most persuasive evidence. In theory, a single, large, well-conducted and controlled clinical trial could provide sufficient evidence to establish a substance and disease relationship.

Interventional studies for foods may differ from those for drugs. Unlike drug studies, food interventional trials may have additional confounders secondary to using a food substance as the intervention. In addition, it may not be possible to use a placebo control group for food studies and subjects in such studies may not be blinded to the intervention. As a result of the greater likelihood for confounders and bias, interventional studies with foods may generate data that has less certainty than data from drug interventional studies.

Although interventional studies are the most reliable category of studies for determining cause-and-effect relationships, generalizing from selected populations often presents serious problems in the interpretation of such studies. Furthermore, in some cases, such as with cancers of different sites, interventional dietary studies are not feasible because diseases with lower frequency of occurrence, such as rare forms of cancer, require very large study samples to detect an effect. Therefore, the scientific evidence supporting a substance/disease relationship may have to be derived wholly or in part from observational studies.

There is no universally valid method for weighing categories of studies. However, in general, observational studies include, in descending order of persuasiveness, cohort (longitudinal) studies, case-control studies, cross-sectional studies, uncontrolled case series or cohort studies, time-series studies, ecological or cross-population studies, descriptive epidemiology, and case reports. Observational studies may be prospective or retrospective. In prospective studies, investigators recruit subjects and observe them prior to the occurrence of the outcome. In retrospective studies, investigators review the records of subjects and interview subjects after the outcome has occurred. Retrospective studies are usually considered to be more vulnerable to bias and measurement error but are less likely to suffer from the subject selection bias that may occur in prospective studies.

Cohort studies compare the outcome of subjects who have received a specific exposure with the outcome of subjects who have not received that exposure. In case-control studies, subjects with the disease are compared to subjects who do not have the disease (control group). Subjects are enrolled based on their outcome rather than based on their exposure. In cross-sectional studies, at a single point in time the number of individuals with a disease who have received a specific exposure is compared to the number of individuals without the disease who did not receive the exposure. Uncontrolled case series studies depict outcomes in a group without comparing to a control group. Time-series studies compare outcomes during different time periods, e.g., whether the rate of occurrence of a particular outcome during one five-year period changed during a subsequent five-year period. In ecological studies, the rate of a disease is compared across different populations. Investigators seek to identify traits of the populations that may cause the disease. Descriptive epidemiology refers to study designs that assess parameters related to the frequency and distribution of disease in a population, such as the leading cause of death. Case reports describe observations of a single or a small number of subjects.

A common weakness of observational studies is the limited ability to ascertain the actual food or nutrient intake for the population studied. Observational data are also generally restricted to identifying associations between food substances and health outcomes, rather than the cause of the relationship.

Research synthesis studies: The role of "research synthesis" studies, including meta-analysis, in the review of data for health claims is as yet unresolved. The appropriateness of such analytical techniques to establish substance/disease relationships is not known. This is especially true when observational data are entered into meta-analyses. Discussions on the topic have been published and there are on-going efforts to identify criteria and critical factors to consider in both conducting and using such analyses, but standardization of this methodology is still emerging. Therefore, in general, such analyses serve as supporting evidence rather than as primary evidence. While meta-analyses have been reviewed as part of the health claim authorization process, no health claims have been authorized on the basis of meta-analysis studies alone[325]. Pharmacoepidemiology is relatively a new branch that uses all the available evidence including that of traditional use or practice along with other types of controlled interventional evidences.

Although human studies are weighted most heavily in the evaluation of evidence on a diet/disease relationship, data from animal model and *in vitro* laboratory studies also can be used to support a substance/disease relationship. Howver, without any data from human studies, animal and *in vitro* studies alone would not adequately support a diet and disease association. Animal and in vitro studies should be considered when there are problems designing interventional studies or in the absence of an appropriate biomarker. If such studies are used, they are subjected to the same kind of assessment as the human studies. The strongest laboratory evidence would be based on data derived from studies on appropriate animal models that have been reproduced in different laboratories, and that give a statistically significant dose-response relationship.

---

[325] Hasselblad V, Mosteller F, Littenberg B, Chalmers TC, Hunick MG, Turner JA, *et. al.*, A survey of current problems in meta-analysis. Discussion from the Agency for Health Care Policy and Research Inter-PORT Work Group on Literature Review/Meta-Analysis. Med Care 1995;33:202-220.

Reliable Measurements

Appropriate measurement is a key factor in the review of data for health claims. Assessing the effects of diet on human health is limited by the use of appropriate biomarkers. A number of the diseases associated with dietary factors are cronic diseases. For example, individuals may have deposits of fat and other material accumulating in the arteries to their hearts leading to athersclerotic/ coronary heart disease yet may not experience any symptoms until years later when they suffer a heart attack. Therefore, scientists seek to identify biomarkers or surrogate markers to predict the presence or risk of disease. A biomarkers is a measurements of a variable related to a disease that may serve as a predictor of developing that disease rather than being a measure of the disease itself. The scientific standard used for the health claim review process does not rely on a change in a biomarker as a measurement of the effect of a dietary factor and a disease unless there is evidence that altering the parameter can affect the risk of developing that disease or health-related condition. This is the case for serum cholesterol in that high levels are generally accepted as a predictor of risk for coronary heart disease and there is evidence that decreasing high serum cholesterol can decrease that risk. Therefore, the evaluation of whether decreasing the intake of dietary fat reduces the risk of developing heart disease took into account many studies that assessed changes in serum cholesterol, specifically LDL-cholesterol, rather the development of heart disease per se. For the existing authorized health claims, acceptable biomarkers are LDL-cholesterol levels for coronary heart disease, measures of bone mass for osteoporosis, and measures of blood pressure for hypertension.

The measurement of a food substance relates to what was measured and how does the measured substance relate to the subject of the health claim. Common difficulties involve separating the effect of the food substance from the food itself, or the use of measures that reflect heterogeneous or poorly defined food substances. Without evidence that the substance, rather than the overall diet or specific foods in the diet, is responsible for the benefit, the linkage between the substance and the disease cannot be established.

During evaluations of the initial 10 substance / disease relationships in 1990-1992, this principle was used. In the case of claims related to omega-3 fatty acids, fiber, and antioxidant vitamins, there was considerable measurement overlap between the food containing the substance and the substance itself, or there were concomitant changes in other dietary components. Both folic acid and fiber were poorly defined and/or heterogeneous mixtures as measured in research available at the time of the initial health claim review. For example, as noted during the health claim authorization process for fiber and heart disease, the objective of the protocols of many studies was to evaluate the effectiveness of relatively large amounts of a single type of food or fiber source rich in soluble fiber rather than to examine total soluble dietary fiber intakes or to specifically identify the chemical and physical characteristics of soluble fiber that are most effective in lowering blood cholesterol levels. While a food can be the subject of a health claim, existing experience is that the subject is more likely to be a group of foods, such as fruits, vegetables, and grains, which have been associated with a reduced risk of heart disease and of cancer. It would be possible that a unique combination of nutrients or other substances in a single food could be the subject of a health claim.

Attention must be given to measurement of dietary intake in the studies reviewed. Each method has its strengths and weaknesses. No one method is adequate for every purpose. Dietary intake assessment methods include food records, 24-hour recalls, and diet histories. Food records are based on the premise that food weights provide an accurate estimation of food intake. Subjects weigh the foods they consume and record those values. Diet histories use questionnaires or interviewers to estimate the typical diet of subjects over a certain period of time.

Evaluation of Individual Studies

The evaluation of study design, protocol, measurement, and statistical issues for individual studies serves as the starting point from which the overall strengths and weaknesses of the data will be determined and the weight of the evidence assessed.

The review of individual studies on substance/disease relationships is standardized as much as possible and generally follows the approaches outlined in the Guide to Clinical Preventive Services[326] and Diet and Health[327].

The persuasiveness of a study depends on the quality of the study. Evaluation of the quality of individual studies on substance and disease relationships begins with a consideration of the inherent strengths and weaknesses of various study designs. The three most important measures of the quality of a study are design, conduct, and analysis and interpretation. Certain study designs tend to be more persuasive because they are less subject to bias and measurement error. The susceptibility of research data to bias and confounding depends on several factors including

---

[326] National Research Council. Diet and Health: Implications for Reducing Chronic Disease Risk. Washington, DC: National Academy Press, 1989.

[327] Department of Health and Human Services, Office of Disease Prevention and Health Promotion. Report of the US Preventive Services Task Force: Guide to Clinical Preventive Services. 2nd ed. Washington, DC: Office of Public Health and Science, April, 1989.

the methods used to choose subjects and to measure outcomes, the use of a comparison (control) group, and whether the study was conducted retrospectively or prospectively. Confounders are factors associated with the disease in question and the intervention, but do not cause the measured outcome.

Several aspects of substance/disease relationships may give rise to confounders. Foods are rarely composed of a simple mixture of chemical constituents. The addition of a nutrient to a diet, or an increase in total daily intake of that nutrient, may have unintended effects. The added nutrient may displace other nutrients in the diet. Therefore, it may be difficult to ascertain whether the health outcome is the result of the added nutrient or the related changes on the original diet. For example, "total diet" was a confounder in a number of studies used to support a claim that lowering of dietary saturated fat intake and resultant decreases in serum LDL-cholesterol led to a reduced risk of coronary heart disease. Other potential confounders include variability in the quantity or quality of the food substance being administered.

Assessment of the quality of individual studies of substance/disease relationships must consider multiple criteria. Adequacy and clarity of the design seeks assurance that the specific questions to be answered by the study were clearly described at the outset. The methodology used in the study must clearly describe and provide appropriate answers to the questions posed by the study. The duration of the study intervention or follow-up period should be sufficient to detect an effect on the outcome of interest. The potential confounding factors need to be identified, assessed, and/or controlled. The subject leaving the study before its completion is properly assessed and a reasonable explanation is provided.

The sample size should be sufficiently large to provide statistical power to conclude the presence or absence of an effect. The demographic factors such as age, gender distribution, race, socioeconomic status, geographic location, family history, health status, and motivation are considered. The inclusion and exclusion criteria of study subjects should be clearly stated. The recruitment procedures to minimize selection bias should be used. For controlled interventions, the subjects must be randomized and should match with demographic and other variables used between control and treatment groups. The randomization should ensure similar control and intervention groups.

The analytical methodology and quality control procedures used to assess dietary intake need to be adequate and the dietary intervention or exposure should be well defined and appropriately measured. Appropriate lead-in period is important, since changes in the diet may induce compensatory metabolic changes and the effect of an intervention should be measured after stabilization or a lead-in period has occurred. In studies with cross-over designs, an appropriate wash-out period should be provided. The dosage form and setting of the intervention should be representative of the real world. Other possible concurrent changes in diet or health-related behavior (weight loss, exercise, alcohol intake, smoking cessation) during the study should be identified, assessed, and/or controlled. The health, intermediate, or surrogate biomarker outcomes need to be appropriately defined and measured and their relevance to health outcomes should be validated. Although foods are generally considered safe (GrAS), extracting or concentrating a food or herbal substance may render it injurious to health.

Ensuring appropriate statistical analyses of the data remains vital. The statistical significance must be interpreted appropriately. It is advised that the individual studies are summarized by means of summary tables. This organizes and guides the comprehensive review and assists in making the process of authorizing a health claim more transparent.

Totality of the Evidence

It is general principle that the totality of the evidence must support the claim. After relevant, good quality studies are identified and their strengths and weaknesses assessed and summarized, a more comprehensive review is conducted based on the body of evidence as a whole. The evaluation of the totality of the evidence providing the basis for the health claim is objective. Conclusions regarding the association between nutritional exposures or interventions and outcomes must be specific to the identified studies and the interpretation limited to the research conducted.

A classic set of reviews that demonstrate the process for evaluating substance/disease relationships is the work conducted by The Task Force on The Evidence Relating Six Dietary Factors to the Nation's Health[328]. The strength of evidence that exposure to a particular food substance is associated with a health outcome depends on several factors. The first consideration in judging the quality of the body of evidence is determining whether most of the evidence is derived from more persuasive classes of study designs. Both the design category and the quality of the research methodology must be considered together. Various coding and scoring schemes have been devised to systematize this process. The U.S. Preventive Services Task Force's grading system assigns a letter code to rate the

[328] Ahrens EH, Connor WE, eds. Symposium: Report of the Task Force on he Evidence Relating Six Dietary Factors to the Nation's Health. Am J Clin Nutr 1979; 23 (suppl): 2621-2748.

quality of the evidence. Other groups have developed systems that score a study quantitatively, assigning points for different aspects of design quality and performance[329]. However, although both study design codes and quantitative scores are appropriate for rating individual studies, they do not adequately describe the evidence as a whole. Another contribution to the strength of the evidence is the number of studies in support of the association. Consistency of results across different settings and types of populations also strengthens an association. In general, the greater the consistency, the more likely a health claim will be authorized. However, repetition of a poorly designed study does not add to the consistency or quality of the evidence. Finally, if the magnitude of the effect is large, yielding strong statistical significance and narrow confidence intervals, evidence of an association is bolstered and the association is more likely to have clinical significance.

Evidence of an association does not, however, prove cause and effect. An association of variables only indicates that they occur together but not that one causes the other. Therefore, another step in the process of a health claim review is to determine the strength of the evidence for a causal relationship. Strength of association, dose-response relationship, and temporal relationship may be used in the evaluation of the totality of the evidence. Although these features strengthen the claim that a substance contributes to a certain health outcome, they do not prove that eating more or less of the substance will produce a clinically meaningful outcome.

---

[329] Mohar D, Jadad AR, Tugwell P. Assessing the quality of randomized controlled trials: current issues and future directions. Int J Technol Assess Health Care 1996;12:125-208.

Relative risk is the ratio between the rate of disease for subjects exposed and not exposed to the substance. Consistency of association means that the same association is found across several studies and among various population groups. Independence of association refers to the extent to which the association relates to the exposure or intervention being studied and the extent to which the association relates to another variable rather than the exposure or intervention. Dose-response relationship requires that greater effects occur with greater exposures to the substance. Temporal relationship means that the exposure should consistently precede the outcome. Effect of dechallenge means that subject from whom the intervention has been withdrawn demonstrate a reversal of the associated outcome. Specificity means that the substance should only be associated with the disease in question. The more specific an association, the more likely the association is causal. In the the comprehensive review, the operative analysis is whether the weight of the evidence supports the existence of a causal relationship between the substance and the disease or health condition that is the subject of a proposed claim.

Scientific Agreement

A significant scientific agreement among qualified experts is necessary before FDA can authorize a health claim. It is important to recognize that significant scientific agreement is not consensus, but it represents considerably more than an initial body of emerging evidence. Significant scientific agreement depends on the strength and consistency of the evidence. Although consensus is not required to demonstrate significant scientific agreement, there is considerable potential for incorrect conclusions if only emerging science is used to authorize health claims.

This is best illustrated by the body of evidence for the association between beta-carotene and cancer risk[330].

The usual mechanism to show that the evidence is available to qualified experts is that the data and information are published in peer-reviewed scientific journals. However, not all the data need be published. Evidence also can be made available through other means, such as scientific meetings. FDA reviews information that is not publicly available as long as that information is placed in the public domain at the time the agency takes action on a health claim petition. When determining whether there is significant agreement, FDA takes into account the viewpoints and opinions of qualified experts outside the agency or recommendation of an authoritative body such as the National Academy of Sciences (NAS), the Committee on Nutrition of the American Academy of Pediatrics (AAP), the American Heart Association (AHA), NIH task forces, and others.

Pharmacoepidemiology

Pharmacology is the study of the effect of drugs and clinical pharmacology is the study of effect of drugs in humans. Part of the task of clinical pharmacology is to provide a risk benefit assessment for the effect of drugs in patients. Doing the studies needed to provide an estimate of the probability of beneficial effects in populations, or the probability of adverse effects in populations and other parameters relating to drug use may benefit from using epidemiological methodology. Thus, Pharmacoepidemiology may be defined as the application

---

[330] Albanes D, Heinonen OP, Huttunen JK, Taylor PR, Virtamo J, Edwards BK, Haapakoski J, Rautalahti M, Hartman AM, Palmgren J, *et. al.*, Effects of alpha-tocopherol and beta-carotene supplements on cancer incidence in the Alpha-Tocopherol Beta-Carotene Cancer Prevention Study. Am J Clin Nutr 1995;62(6 Suppl):1427S-1430S.

of epidemiological methods to pharmacological issues[331]. Epidemiology is the study of the distribution and determinants of diseases in populations. Epidemiological studies are divided into two main types: Descriptive and Analytical. Descriptive epidemiology involves study of diseases, exposure and their rates, e.g., incidence and prevalence. Studies of drug utilization generally fall under this. Analytic epidemiology includes two types of studies: observational studies, which include case-control and cohort studies; and experimental studies, which include randomized Phase 1 - 4 clinical trials. The analytic studies compare exposed groups with a control groups and are normally designed as hypothesis testing studies in open label, single or double blind studies. Pharmacoepidemiology thus is a bridge science overlapping both pharmacology and epidemiology and involves study of the utilization and effects of drugs in large numbers of people[332]. Pharmacoepidemiology benefits from the epidemiology methodology and develop them for applications to some areas like pharmacovigilance. Although these are relatively new branches, already formal associations such as International Society for Pharmacoepidemiology (ISPE) are already active. Pharmacovigilance involves continual monitoring for unwanted effects and other safety-related aspects of marketed drugs. Pharmacovigilance refers to the spontaneous reporting systems, which allow health care professionals and others to report adverse drug reactions to a central agency. The central agency can then combine reports from many sources to produce a more informative safety profile for the drug product than could be done based

---

[331] Hartzema A.G., Porta M. Tilson, M, H.H. Editors. - An Introduction to Pharmacoepidemiology, 1998 Third Edition. Harvey Whitney Books Company.

[332] Strom, B.L. Editor. Pharrmacoepidemiology, 2000, Third Edition, John Wiley & Sons.

on one or a few reports from one or a few health care professionals.

Pharmacoepidemiology and Pharmacovigilance are important in ethnopharmacology and drug discovery for systematic documenting the evidence base arising from traditional use of different medicines. Here the process is reversed as the drugs are already in market and are consumed for sufficiently number of people for a long time. Hence most of the observational and experiencial information about its efficacy, safety or toxicity is available. Traditional medical systems such as Ayurveda have evidence of practice and use and if systematically compiled and statistically analyzed could give a fair evidence base. Recently, a new branch called Ayurvedic pharmacoepidemiology has been proposed to apply epidemiological and statistical methods for traditional practice data to organize and analyze it for consideration of scientific and regulatory authorities[333].

❑❑❑

[333] Vaidya Rama *et. al.*, Ayurvedic Pharmacoepidemiology, Journal of Association of Physicians of India, 2004.

Part III : Technology

12 Biotechnology in Herbal Drug Research

The main purpose of herbal drug technology is to convert botanical materials into medicines with a focus on standardization and quality control with proper integration of modern scientific techniques and traditional knowledge. The use of chromatographic techniques and marker compounds to standardize botanical preparations has limitations because of their variable sources and chemical complexity. DNA-based molecular markers have utility in fields like taxonomy, physiology, embryology, genetics etc. DNA based techniques have widely been used for authentication of plant species of medicinal importance. Pharmacognosy mainly addresses the quality related issues using routine botanical and organoleptic parameters of crude drugs, and chemoprofiling assisted characterization with chromatographic and spectroscopic techniques. The new pharmacognosy includes all the aspects of drug development and discovery where the biotechnology driven applications play an important role. Current focus on chemotype-driven fingerprinting and related techniques require integration with genotype-driven molecular techniques so that an optimal characterization of botanical materials is possible. This review provides a brief account of various DNA based technologies that are useful in genotyping and quick identification of botanicals with suitable examples.

Current Trends in Herbal Medicine

Use of indigenous drugs from plant origin forms a major part of the Complimentary and Alternative Medicine/ Traditional Medicine (CAM/TM). The world market for herbal medicine including herbal products and raw materials has been estimated to have an annual growth rate between 5 to 15 %. Total global herbal drug market is estimated as US $62 billion and is expected to grow to US $5 trillion by the year 2050[334]. India has a great wealth of traditional knowledge and wisdom. Ayurveda contributes Rs 3500 crores (US $813 Million) annually to the internal market. The Indian medicinal plants based industry is growing at the rate of 7-15% annually. The value of medicinal plants related trade in India is estimated at Rs 5,000 crores annually. Global trends leading to increased demands of medicinal plants for pharmaceuticals, phytochemicals, nutraceuticals, cosmetics and other products is an opportunity for Indian trade and commerce[335]. Scientifically validated and technologically standardized herbal medicines may be derived using the reverse pharmacology approach based on an existing traditional knowledge database[336]. This may play a vital role in drug discovery, development and therapeutics in addition to dealing with a typical western bias against Ayurveda[337]. Herbal drug technology includes all the steps

[334] Report of the Inter Regional Workshop on Intellectual Property Rights in the Context of Traditional Medicine, Bangkok, Thailand, December 2000.

[335] Singh, J., Singh, A. K. and Khanuja, S. P. S., Pharma Bio World, 2003, 1(3), 59-66

[336] Vaidya A.D.B., Vaidya R.A., Nagaral S.I. J. Assoc. Phys. India, 2001, 49, 534-537.

[337] Patwardhan B., Chopra A., Vaidya A.D.B. Current Science, 2003, 84 (9), 1165-1166.

that are involved in converting botanical materials into medicines where standardization and quality control with proper integration of modern scientific techniques and traditional knowledge will remain important. Herbal medicinal products may vary in composition and properties, unlike conventional pharmaceutical products, which are usually prepared from synthetic, chemically pure materials by means of reproducible manufacturing techniques and procedures. Correct identification and quality assurance of the starting material is, therefore, an essential prerequisite to ensure reproducible quality of herbal medicine, which contributes to its safety and efficacy[338,339].

Methods of Identification, Limitations and Emerging Techniques

Most of the regulatory guidelines and pharmacopoeias suggest macroscopic and microscopic evaluation and chemical profiling of the botanical materials for quality control and standardization[340,341,9]. Macroscopic identity of botanical materials is based on parameters like shape, size, color, texture, surface characteristics, fracture characteristics, odor, taste and such organoleptic properties that are compared to a standard reference material. Microscopy involves comparative microscopic inspection of broken as well as powdered crude botanical materials. However, these parameters are judged subjectively and substitutes or adulterants may closely resemble the genuine

---

[338] Straus S.E., New Engl. J. Med., 2002, 347, 1997-1998.

[339] De Smet PAGM, N Engl J Med., 2002, 347 (25), 2046-2056.

[340] Indian Herbal Pharmacopoeia, Indian Drug Manufacturers' Association, Mumbai, 2002.

[341] British Herbal Pharmacopoeia, British Herbal Medicine Association, 1996.

material. Chemical profiling establishes a characteristic chemical pattern for a plant material, its fractions or extracts. Thin-layer chromatography (TLC) and High performance thin layer chromatography (HPTLC) are routinely used as valuable tools for the qualitative determination of small amounts of impurities. In addition, many analytical techniques such as volumetric analysis, gravimetric determinations, gas chromatography, column chromatography, high performance liquid chromatography, and spectrophotometric methods are also frequently used for quality control and standardization[342].

The use of chromatographic techniques and marker compounds to standardize botanical preparations has limitations because of their variable sources and chemical complexity. The variability in the flavors, aroma, physical characteristics of wine and coffee from year to year and region to region provide a good analogy. Many factors may affect the ultimate chemical profile of any herb. Intrinsic factors such as genetics and extrinsic factors such as cultivation, harvesting, drying and storage conditions are few examples[343]. The routine chemotaxonomic studies provide only a qualitative account of secondary metabolites. For quantitative studies, use of specific markers that can be easily analyzed to distinguish between varieties, remains the preferred option. Using such metabolites as markers may or may not be therapeutically active but should ideally be neutral to environmental effects and management practices[344].

---

[342] Quality Control Methods for Medicinal Plant Materials, WHO, Geneva, 1998.

[343] An Exploration of Current Issues in Botanical Quality: A Discussion Paper , Natural Health Products Directorate, Health Products and Food Branch, Canada, February 2002.

[344] Joshi, S. P., Ranjekar, P. K., and Gupta, V. S., Curr. Sci., 1999, 77, 230-240.

In order to ensure efficacy, selection of the correct chemotype of the plant is necessary. Even when there are many known chemotypes of a plant species, selection of the right chemotype to which clinical effects are attributed is difficult. For example, *Withania somnifera* is reported to have three chemotypes depending upon the presence of class of closely related steroidal lactones like Withanolides, Withaferin A etc. The content of Withanolides and Withaferin A and other biologically active compounds may vary depending upon the environment, genotype, time of collection of plant material etc. Hence selection of the right chemotype is important to therapeutic efficacy[345].

Another difficulty encountered in the selection of the correct plant material is to establish the identity of certain species that may be known by different binomial botanical names in different regions. For example, Shankhapushpi which is an important medhya Rasayan in Ayurveda is equated with one or other of the following plants depending upon the region in India: *Canscora decussata, Evolvulus alsinoides* and *Clitoria ternata*[346]. Certain rare and expensive medicinal plant species are often adulterated or substituted by morphologically similar, easily available or less expensive species. For example *Swertia chirata* is frequently adulterated or substituted by the cheaper *Andrographis paniculata*[347].

In light of these limitations, there is need for a new approach that can complement or in certain situations serve as an alternative. Some of the newly emerging techniques for ensuring correct botanical identity and quality include Herboprint™, which in addition to chemoprofile also

[345] Bhutani, K. K., The Eastern Pharmacist, 2000, 21-26.

[346] Rao, E. V., The Eastern Pharmacist, 2000, 35-38.

[347] Sri Bhava Misra., Bhavaprakash (ed. Misra, B. and Vaisya, R.), Chaukhambha Sanskrit Sansthan, Varanasi, 1999,vol.1, pp.73-75.

considers Ayurvedic properties[348] and capillary electrophoresis. This technique is a faster, precise and sensitive method and has recently been used to ascertain the botanical identity and quality of *Ephedrae herba*[349], *Coptidis rhizoma*[350], *Ginseng radix*[351] and *Paeoniae radix*[352].

Molecular markers generally refer to biochemical constituents including primary and secondary metabolites and other macromolecules such as nucleic acids. Secondary metabolites as markers have been extensively used in quality control and standardization of botanical drugs. We are focusing the present review only on DNA markers, which may have several advantages over typical phenotype markers. DNA markers are reliable markers for informative polymorphisms because the genetic composition is unique for each species and is less affected by age, physiological conditions as well as environmental factors[353]. DNA can be extracted from fresh or dried organic tissue of the botanical material; hence the physical form of the sample for assessment does not restrict detection. Various DNA based methods for species characterization and adulteration detection in medicinal plants; agricultural crops and genetically modified (GM) foods have been published.

---

[348] Vijaya Kumar,D. and Raghavan, K. V., Indian Institute of Chemical Technology, Hyderabad, Novel Chromatographic fingerprinting method for standardization of single medicines and formulations.,WO 0246739-EP2 0000991 991-263397CSIR G01N30-88.

[349] Liu, Y. M., Sheu, S. J., Chiou, S.H., Chang, S. H. and Chen, Y. P., Planta Med., 1993,59,376-378.

[350] Liu, Y. M., Sheu, S. J., Chiou, S.H., Chang, S. H. and Chen, Y. P., Phytochem. Anal., 1994, 5, 256-260.

[351] Chuang, W. C., Wu, S. K., Sheu, S. J., Chiou, S. H., Chang, H. C. and Chen, Y. P., Planta Med., 1995,61, 459-465.

[352] Chuang, W. C., Wu, S. K., Sheu, S. J., Chiou, S. H., Chang, H. C. and Chen, Y. P., Planta Med., 1996,62, 459-465.

[353] Chan, K., Chemosphere, 2003, 52, 1361-1371.

Types of DNA Markers Used in Plant Genome Analysis

Various types of DNA based molecular markers are utilized to evaluate DNA polymorphism and are generally classified as hybridization-based markers, Polymerase Chain Reaction (PCR)-based markers and sequencing based markers.

Hybridization-Based Markers

Hybridization-based markers include Restriction Fragment Length Polymorphism (RFLP) and Variable Number Tandem Repeats (VNTR) loci where probes such as random genomic clones, cDNA clones, probes for microsatellite and minisatellite sequences are hybridized to filters containing DNA which has been digested with restriction enzymes.

PCR-Based Markers

These are fingerprinting techniques that use the polymerase chain reaction (PCR) to specifically amplify a multiplicity of target sites in one or more nucleic acid molecules (Caetano-Anollés 1996, Micheli and Bova 1996). PCR-based markers can be random or specific depending upon the type of primer used, the stringency of the PCR conditions and the method of fragment separation and detection. Random PCR markers include Random Amplified Polymorphic DNA (RAPD), Arbitrarily Primed PCR (AP-PCR) and DNA Amplification Fingerprinting (DAF). Specific PCR-based markers include Inter Simple Sequence Repeats (ISSRs) which is a PCR based marker for genome analysis where a terminally anchored primer specific to a particular SSR is used to amplify the DNA between two opposed SSRs of the same type. A recent approach known as Amplified Fragment Length Polymorphism (AFLP) is a technique that is based on the detection of genomic restriction fragments by PCR amplification and can be used for DNAs of any origin or complexity[354].

Sequencing -Based Markers

DNA sequencing is a definitive means for identifying TCM. Further, variation due to transversion, insertion or deletion can be assessed directly and information on a defined locus can be obtained.

Applications of Molecular Markers in Herbal Drug Technology

DNA based molecular markers have proved their utility in fields like taxonomy, physiology, embryology, genetics etc. As the science of plant genetics progressed researchers have tried to explore these molecular marker techniques for their applications in commercially important plants such as food crops, horticultural plants, etc. and recently in pharmacognostic characterization of herbal medicine.

Genetic variation / Genotyping

It has been well documented that geographical conditions affect the active constituents of the medicinal plant and hence their activity profiles[355]. Many researchers have studied geographical variation at the genetic level. Estimates of genetic diversity are also important in designing crop improvement programmes, for management of germplasm and evolving conservation strategies. RAPD based molecular markers have been found to be useful in differentiating different accessions of *Taxus wallichiana*[356],

---

[354] Kumar, L. S., Biotechnology Advances.,1999,17, 143-182.

[355] Oleszek, W., Stochmal, A., Karolewski, P., Simonet, A.M., Macias, F.A. and Tava, A., Biochem Syst Ecol., 2002, 30(11), 1011-1022.

[356] Shasany, A. K., Kukreja, A. K.,Saikia, D., Darokar, M. P., Khanuja, S. P. S. and Kumar, S., PGR Newsletter, 1999,121, 27-31.

neem[357], *Juniperus communis* L.[358], *Codonopsis pilosula*[359], *Allium schoenoprasum* L.[360], *Andrographis paniculata*[361] collected from different geographical regions. Similarly, different accessions of *Cannabis sativa*[362] have been discriminated using ISSR markers and those of *Arabidopsis thaliana* L. Heynh.[363] have been differentiated using Cleaved Amplified Polymorphic Sequence (CAPS) and ISSR markers. Inter and intraspecies variation has also been studied using DNA based molecular markers. Interspecies variation has been studied using RFLP and RAPD in different genus such as *Glycerrhiza*[364], *Echinacea*[365], *Curcuma*[366] and *Arabidopsis*[367]. RAPD and RFLP have also been applied for characterization of *Epimedium*[368] species at the genetic level. Members of three different species of *Scutellaria*[369], Chinese medicinal plants and three subspecies

---

[357] Farooqui, N., Ranade, S. A. and Sane, P. V., Biochem Mol Biol Int., 1998, 45 (5), 931-939.

[358] Adams, R.P., Pandeyb, R. N.,Leverenzc, J. W., Digdardd, N., Hoeghe, K. and Thorfinnssonf, T., Scientia Horticulturae, 2002,96 (1-4), 303-312.

[359] Fu, R. Z., Wang, J., Zhang, Y. B., Wang, Z. T., But, P. P., Li, N. and Shaw, P. C., Planta med, 1999,65(7), 648-650.

[360] Friesen, N.and Blattner, F. R., Planta med., 1999, 65, 157-160.

[361] Padmesh, P., Sabu, K.K. and Seeni, S., and Pushpangadan, P., Curr Sci., 76 (6), 833-835.

[362] Kojoma, M., Iida, O., Makino, Y., Sekita, S. and Satake, M., Planta med, 2002, 68 (1), 60-63.

[363] Barth, S., Melchinger, A. E., Lubberstedt, T., Mol Ecol., 2002,11(3), 495-505.

[364] Yamazaki, M., Sato, A., Shimomura, K., Saito, K. and Murakoshi, I., Biol Pharm Bull, 1994, 17 (11), 529-1531.

[365] Kapteyn, J.,Goldsbrough, B. and Simon, E., Theor Appl genet., 2002, 105(2-3), 369-376.

[366] Chen, Y., Bai, S., Cheng, K., Zhang, s. and Nian L., Zhongguo Zhong Yao Za Zhi., 1999, 24(3), 131-133.

[367] Lind-Hallden, C., Hallden, C. and Sall, T., Hereditas, 2002, 136 (1), 45-50.

[368] Nakai, R., Shoyama, Y. and Shiraishi, S., Biol. Pharm Bull., 1996,19 (1), 67-70.

[369] Hosokawa, K., Minami, M., Kawahara, K., Nakamura, I. and Shibata, T., Planta med., 2000, 66 (3), 270-272.

of *Melissa officinalis*[370] have been discriminated using RAPD. Varietal characterization of Kenaf (*Hibiscus cannabinus* L.)[371] has been done with the help of agronomical and RAPD data. Varietal identification and genetic purity test in Pepper and *Capsicum annuum* were carried out using RAPD markers[372]. RFLP technique was used for interspecific genetic variation within the genus Capsicum and also for DNA fingerprinting of pepper cultivars[373]. RAPD has served as a tool for the detection of variability in Jojoba (*Simmondsia chinensis* L. Schneider)[374], *Vitis vinifera* L.[375] and in tea (*Camellia sinesis*)[376]. Attempts have been made to understand the population structure of *Podophyllum peltatum* to establish commercial level propagation of useful secondary metabolites using molecular markers[377]. Also, high genetic diversity has been shown in *Podophyllum hexandrum* species from Himachal Pradesh, India[378]. Genetic variation and relationships among and within *Withania* species[379] and genetic relationships among Papaya and its wild relatives

---

[370] Wolf, H. T., Berg, T. V. D., Czygan, FC., Mosandl, A., Winckler, T., Zundorf, I. and Dingermann, T., Planta Med, 1999, 65, 83-85.

[371] Cheng, Z., Lu, B. R., Baldwin, B. S., Sameshima, K. and Chen, J. K., Hereditas, 2002, 136 (3), 231-239

[372] Hulya, I., Scientia Horticulturae, 2003, 97 (3-4), 211-218.

[373] Prince, J. P., Lackney, V. K., Angels, C., Blauth, J. R. and Kyle, M. M., Genome, 1995, 38(2), 224-231

[374] Amarger, V. and Mercier, L., Biochimie, 1995, 72 (12), 931-936.

[375] Tessier,C., David, J., this, P., Boursiquot, J. M. and Charrier, A., Theor Appl Genet, 1999, 98, 171-177.

[376] Wachira, F. N., Waugh, R., Hackett, C. A and Powell, W., Genome, 1995, 38 (2), 201-210.

[377] Lata, H., Moraes, R. M., Douglas, A. and Scheffler, B. E., Trends in new crops and new uses (eds. Janick, J. and Whipkey, A.), ASHS Press, alexandria, VA, 2002, pp. 537-539.

[378] Singh, B. M., Sharma, K. D., Katoch, M., Guleria, S. and Sharma, T. R., PGR newsletter, 1999, 124, 57-61.

[379] Negi, M. S., Singh, A. and Laksmikumaran, M., Genome,2000, 43, 975-80.

(*Caricaceae*)[380] have been revealed using AFLP markers. Genetic variation within *Brassica campestris* cultivars has been studied using AFLP and RAPD markers[381].

Phylogenetic relationships between citrus and its relatives have been studied using SSR markers[382]. RAPD has been used to construct genetic linkage maps of *Eucalyptus grandis* and *Eucalyptus urophylla*[383]. RAPD markers have been developed for genetic mapping of Pacific yew (*Taxus bravifolia* Nutt.)[384]. An attempt has been made to develop a physical AFLP map of the complex *Arabidopsis* genome by combining gel-based AFLP analysis with *in silico* restriction fragment analysis using the published genome sequence[385].

Authentication of Medicinal Plants

DNA based techniques have widely been used for authentication of plant species of medicinal importance. This is especially useful in case of those that are frequently substituted or adulterated with other species or varieties that are morphologically and/or phytochemically indistinguishable.

Dried fruit samples of *Lycium barbarum* were differentiated from its related species using RAPD

---

380 Van, DB, Breyne P., Goetghebeur, P, Romijn-Peeters, E, Kyndt,T and Gheysen, G., Theor Appl Genet, 2002, 105 (2-3), 289-297.

381 Das, S., Rajagopal, J., Bhatia, S., Srivastava, P. S. and Lakshmikumaran, M., J. Biosci., 1999, 24(4), 233-240.

382 Pang, X. M., Hu, C. G. and Deng, X. X., Yi chuan Xue Bao, 2003, 30 (1), 81-87.

383 Grattapaglia, D. and Sederoff, R., Genetics, 1994,137,1121-1137.

384 Gocmen, B., Jermstad, K. D., Neale, D. B. and Kaya, Z., Can. J. For. Res., 1996, 26, 497-503.

385 Peters, J. L., Constandt, H., Neyt, P., Cnops, G., Zethof, J., Zabeau, M. and Gerats, T., Plant Physiol., 2001, 127(4),1579-1589.

markers[386]. RAPD technique has also been used to determine the components of a Chinese herbal prescription, yu-ping-feng san. In this study, the presence of three herbs (*Astragalus membanaceus* (Fisch.) Bge., *Ledebouriella seseloides* Wolff, and *Atractylodes macrocephala* Koidz) in the formulation have been detected using a single RAPD primer[387].

Three RAPD primers have been identified that could successfully discriminate between three species of *Atractylodes*, from Chinese formulation purchased in local markets[388]. In another study, three random primers were used to reveal the genetic variability of *Astragalus* medicine materials sold in Taiwan market. SSCP analysis was also conducted on PCR products from the ITS-1 region of ribosomal DNA in order to differentiate the two *Astragalus* species[389]. Primers have been designed for hybridization with the hypervariable ends of microsatellite loci that could reveal DNA-polymorphisms among five Eucalyptus species[390]. DAF has been used to distinguish the Chinese traditional medicine, *Magnoliae officinalis*, from its counterfeits and substitutes[391]. A RAPD primer that is selective for an elite strain Aizu K-111 of *Panax ginseng*

---

[386] Zhang, K. Y., Leung, H. W., Yeung, H.W. and Wong, R. N., Planta med., 2001, 67 (4), 379-381.

[387] Cheng, K. T., Tsay, H. S., Chen, C. F. and Chou, T. W., Planta med., 1998, 64 (6), 563-565.

[388] Chen, K. T., Su, Y. C., Lin, J. G., Hsin, L. H., Su, Y. P., Su, C. H., Li, S. Y., Cheng, J. H. and Mao, S. J., Acta Pharmacol Sin, 2001, 22, 493-497.

[389] Cheng , K. T., Su, B., Chen, C. T. and Lin, C. C., Am J Chin Med., 2000, 28 (2), 273-278.

[390] Matsuda,M., Kojima, E., Izumi, M.,Murakami, K., Nucleic Acids Symp Ser., 1997 ,37, 169-170.

[391] Wang, T., Su, Y., Zhu, J., Li, X., Zeng, O. and Xia, N. Zhong Yao Cai, 2001, 24(10), 710-715.

including its cultured tissues has been identified [392]. RAPD and PCR-RFLP analysis have been used for authentication of *Panax ginseng* among ginseng populations[393]. Some researchers have used a new approach called Direct Amplification of Length Polymorphism (DALP) for authentication of *Panax ginseng* and *Panax quinquefolius*[394].

Detection of Adulteration or Substitution

RAPD technique was adopted to identify eight types of dried *Coptis* rhizomes and one type of *Picrorrhiza* rhizome, a substitute for the former in the Chinese herbal market[395]. *Panax ginseng* is often substituted by *P. quinquefolius* (American ginseng). SCAR, AP-PCR, RAPD and RFLP markers have been successfully applied for differentiation of these plants and to detect substitution by other closely related species[396,397,398]. Characterization of *Echinacea* species and detection of possible adulterations has been done by using RAPD technique[399]. DNA fingerprinting and polymorphism in the Chinese drug "Ku-Di-Dan" (herba elephantopi) and its substitutes were studied using AP-PCR and RAPD. The results were used for authentication of "Ku-

[392] Yukiko, T. K., Asaka., I. And Ichio, I., Biol. Pharm. Bull., 2001, 24 (10), 1210-1213.

[393] Um, J. Y., Xchung, H. S., Kim, M. S., Na, H. J., et al. Biol. Pharm. Bull., 2001, 24 (8), 872-875.

[394] Ha, W. Y., Yau, F. C., But, P. P., Wang, J. and Shaw, P. C., Planta med, 2001, 67 (6), 587-589.

[395] Cheng, K. T., Chang, H. C., Su, C. H. and Hsu, F. L., Bot. Bull. Acad. Sin., 1997, 38, 241-244.

[396] Shaw, P. C. and But, P. P., Planta med., 1995, 61 (5),466-469.

[397] Wang, J., Ha, W. Y., Ngan, F. N., But, P. P. H. and Shaw, P. C., Planta med., 2001, 67,781-783.

[398] Mihalov, J. J., Marderosian, A. D. and Pierce, J. C., J Agric Food Chem., 2000, 48 (8), 3744-3752.

[399] Wolf, H.T., Zundorf, I., Winckler, T., Bauer, R. and Dingermann, T., Planta med., 1999, 65, 773-774.

Di-Dan" and its substitutes[400]. DNA fingerprinting of *Taraxacum mongolicum* (herba taraxaci) and its adulterants of six species of Compositae was demonstrated using AP-PCR and RAPD[401]. Bulb of *Fritillaria cirrhosa,* an official drug of Chinese Pharmacopoeia (1995) is commonly used as an antitussive and expectorant. It has often been adulterated with similar bulbs of other related species. Specific DNA based primers have been designed for authentication of *F. cirrhosa* at the genomic level[402]. A molecular marker that is specific to medicinal Rhubarb based on chloroplast trnL/trnF sequence that is absent in its adulterants has been identified[403].

DNA sequence analysis of rDNA internal transcribed spacer (ITS) and PCR-RFLP were explored for their applications in differentiating four medicinal *Codonopsis* species from their related adulterants, *Campanumoea javania* and *Platycodon grandiflorus*. The technique allowed effective and reliable differentiation of *Codonopsis* from the adulterants.

Marker Assisted Selection of Desirable Chemotypes

Along with authentication of species identity, prediction of the concentration of active phytochemicals may be required for quality control in the use of plant materials for pharmaceutical purposes. Identification of DNA markers that can correlate DNA fingerprinting data with the quantity of selected phytochemical markers

---

[400] Cao, H., But, P. P. and Shaw, P. C., Yao, Xue Xue Bao.,1996, 31 (7), 543-553.

[401] Cao, H., But, P. P. and Shaw, P., Zhongguo Zhong Yao Za Zhi, 1997, 22(4), 197-200.

[402] Li, Y. F., Li, X. Y., Lin, J., Xu, Y., Yan, L., Tang, F. and Chen, F., Planta med, 2003, 69,186-188.

[403] Yang, M., Zhang, D., Liu, J. and Zheng, J., Planta Med., 2001, 67(8), 784-786.

associated with a particular plant would have extensive applications in Quality Control of raw materials. AFLP analysis has been found to be useful in predicting phytochemical markers in cultivated *Echinacea purpurea*[404] germplasm and some related wild species. RAPD fingerprint has been developed to support the chemotypic differences in oil quality of three different genotypes of *Pelargonium graveolens*[405] and flavonoid composition of *Aconitum*[406] species. DNA profiling has been used to detect the phylogenetic relationship among *Acorus calamus* chemotypes, which differ in their essential oil composition[407]. *Artemisia annua,* source of antimalarial compound artemisinin shows variation in artemisinin content all over India. These chemotype variants of *Artemisia annua* L. have been characterized using RAPD markers. This study also revealed existence of very high levels of genetic variation in the Indian population despite geographical isolation, a finding that opens the possibility of further genetic improvement for superior artemisinin content. Attempts have also been made to study variation in essential oil components and interspecific variations using RAPD technique[408]. Morphological, chemical and genetic differences in twelve basil (*Ocimum gratissimum* L.) accessions were studied to determine whether volatile oil and flavonoids can be used as taxonomical markers and to

---

[404] Baum, B. R., Mechanda, S., Livesey, J. F., Binns, S.E. and Arnason, J. T., Phytochemistry, 2001,56,543-549.

[405] Shasany, A. K., Aruna, V., Darokar, M. P., Kalra, A., Bahl, J. R., Bansal, R. P. and Khanuja, S. P. S., J Med Arom Plant Sci., 2002, 24 , 729-732.

[406] Fico, G., Spada, A., Bracab, A., Agradic, E., Morellib, I. and Tomea, F., Biochem Syst Ecol., 2003,31 (3), 293-301.

[407] Sugimoto, N., Kiuchi, F., Mikage, M., Mori, M., Mizukami, H. and Tsuda, Y., Biol Pharm Bull., 1999, 22(5), 481-485.

[408] Sangwan, R. S., Sangwan, N. S., Jain, D. C., Kumar, S.and Ranade, S. A., Biochem Mol Biol Int, 47 (6), 935-944.

examine the relation between RAPDs to these chemical markers[409].

Medicinal Plant Breeding

ISSR-PCR has been found to be a very efficient and reliable technique for the identification of zygotic plantlets in citrus interploid crosses[410]. Molecular markers have been used as a tool to verify sexual and apomictic offspring of intraspecific crosses in *Hypericum perforatum*, a well-known antihelminthic and diuretic[411]. An attempt has been made towards marker-assisted selection of fertile clones of garlic with the help of RAPD markers[412]. RAPD markers have been successively used for selection of micropropogated plants of *Piper longum* for conservation[413].

Applications in Foods and Nutraceuticals

DNA based molecular markers have been used extensively for a wide range of applications in food crops and horticultural plants[409,410,414]. These applications include study of genetic variation, cultivar identification, genotyping, cross breeding studies, identification of disease resistant genes, identification of quantitative trait loci, diversity analysis of exotic germplasms, sex identification of dioeceous plants, phylogenetic analysis, etc.

---

[409] Vieira, R. F., Grayer, R. J., Paton, A. and Simon, J. E., Biochem Syst Ecol., 2001, 29 (3), 287-304.

[410] Tusa, N., Abbet, L., Ferrante, S., Lucreti, S. and Scarano, M. T., Cell Mol Biol Lett, 2002, 7(2B), 703-708.

[411] Steck, N., Messmer, M., Schaffner, W., Bueter, K. B., Plant biol., 2001,622-628.

[412] Etoh, T., Hong, C. J., Acta Horticulturae, 555, II International Symposium on edible Alliaceae.

[413] Parani, M., Anand, A. and Parida, A., Curr Sci., 1997, 73 (1), 81-83.

[414] Sharma, H. C., Crouch, J. H., Sharma, K. K., Seetharama, N. and Hash, C. T., Plant Sci., 2002, 163 (3), 381-395.

Recently, the application of DNA based molecular markers is being explored in the field of nutraceuticals.

According to new European Council (EC) legislation[415], the labeling of food or food ingredients produced from, or containing licensed Genetically Modified Organisms (GMOs) must indicate the inclusion of these ingredients where they are present at or above a level of 1%. In compliance with the labeling regulation for GM foods, several countries in Europe such as Germany and Switzerland have extensively developed PCR methods for both identification and quantification purposes.

In response to reports of unlicensed GM ingredients in foods on the international market, the Food Safety Authority of Ireland (FSAI) has completed a survey to determine the levels of GM maize ingredients in tortilla chips and taco shells on sale in Ireland using the PCR technique[416]. Where sufficient GM DNA was present in the sample, quantitative analysis was undertaken using Real-Time PCR.

Primers specific for inserted genes in the Roundup Ready™ soybean have been found to be suitable for detection and discrimination of GM soybean from non-GM products[417]. In another study, Roundup Ready Soybeans, Bt 176 maize, and Cecropin D capsicum have been successfully discriminated from non-GM products using primers specific for inserted genes and crop endogenous genes[418].

---

[415] http://europa.eu.int/eur-lex/en/lif/dat/2000/en_300R0049.html

[416] http://www.fsai.ie/industry/tortilla_survey.pdf

[417] Lin, H. Y., Chiang, J. and Shih, D. Y. C.,J. Food and Drug Anal, 2001, 9(3), 160-166.

[418] Deng, P., Zhao, J., Liu, J. and Fang, S., Wei Sheng Yan Jiu., 2002, 31 (1), 37-40.

DNA Markers as a New Pharmacognostic Tool

Traditionally, pharmacognosy mainly addressed the quality related issues using routine botanical and organoleptic parameters of crude drugs. Pharmacognosy became more interdisciplinary because of subsequent advances in analytical chemistry. These developments added emphasis on chemoprofiling assisted characterization with chromatographic and spectroscopic techniques. The new pharmacognosy includes all the aspects of drug development and discovery and it is predicted that biotechnology driven applications will play an important role.

Extensive research on DNA based molecular markers is in progress in many research institutes all over the world. This technique remains very important in plant genome research with its applications in pharmacognostic identification and analysis. Chinese researchers have applied DNA markers extensively for characterization of botanicals from the Chinese Materia Medica. These markers have shown remarkable utility in quality control of commercially important botanicals like *Ginseng, Echinacea,* and *Atractylodes*. In India several agricultural universities and research institutes including National Chemical Laboratory, National Botanical Research Institute, Regional Research Laboratories, Central Institute for Medicinal and Aromatic Plants and such are actively involved in exploring DNA based techniques in genotyping of medicinal plants. Although, considerable progress has been made in DNA marker technology, applications of these techniques for characterizing semi-processed and processed botanical formulations to ensure the desirable quality remains under utilized.

Current focus on chemotype-driven fingerprinting and related techniques require integration with genotype-driven molecular techniques so that an optimal characterization of botanical materials is possible. Further, Ayurvedic classification of medicinal plant is based on basic principles and therapeutic characters that may have a genetic basis. We have undertaken an exploratory study on use of molecular markers for quick identification of botanical materials in crude, semi-processed and processed herbal formulations. Our strategy involves identification of species specific markers after screening a number of species and/or varieties of the medicinal plant using random oligonucleotide primers, followed by cloning and subsequently converting it to SCAR markers for better specificity and reproducibility. Also, application of RAPD markers has been explored for standardization of botanical formulations containing Ayurvedic medicines like *Emblica officinalis*[419], *Tinospora cordifolia*[420].

❑❑❑

[419] Warude, D., DNA fingerprinting: A new pharmacognostic tool in drug development., M Pharm Dissertation, 2003, Faculty of Pharmaceutical Sciences, Bharati Vidyapeeth, Pune.

[420] Patil, M., Chemical and pharmacognostic investigations of Tinospora cordifoloia. Ph. D Thesis, 2003, Faculty of Pharmaceutical Sciences, University of Pune.

13 Microarrays and High Throughput Screening

In the area of pharmaceutical discovery, screening methods continue to play a major role in drug discovery. The screening process is simply testing molecular entities (compounds/natural products) for activity to advance those that exhibit the desired activity. This process has evolved over time in both the testing methods and in the degree of testing. Originally, the screening was done entirely by dosing animals and studying their responses. Then came test tube experiments and now, testing is conducted either with cell lines or with purified proteins in miniaturized test tubes called microplate wells. Screening by microplate has allowed the degree of testing to increase from a very small selected set of compounds to libraries, which contain thousands of test substances. Technological improvements in many areas of science and information technology have led to the evolution of screening methods from time consuming, animal dosing studies to high throughput screening (HTS) methods that have the potential to generate very large datasets of information in a very short time. Today, developments in bioinformatics have opened up the possibility of virtual (*in silico*) screens for targets where there is sufficient knowledge of the target or of its ligand. High throughput screening has become a pivotal part of drug discovery for identifying potential lead molecules for specific disease targets. The success of screening is measured by several factors including the throughput and costs of the assays, but ultimately by how many of the HTS hits progress forward through the drug discovery pipeline. Miniaturization of assays by conversion from 96- to 384- to 1536- wells to well-less platforms, such as microarrays and the utilization of automated equipments are methodologies implemented to increase the throughput and reduce the cost of the screen.

Role of Microarrays

Understanding the functions of genes is a major post genomics challenge. A number of 'omics' strategies like proteomics, transcriptomics, metabolomics, etc are implemented to assign the role of genes in molecular networks. The gene expression profile of a cell determines its phenotype, function, and response to the environment. The complement of genes expressed by a cell is very dynamic and responds rapidly to external stimuli. Therefore, analysis of gene expression becomes necessary for providing clues about regulatory mechanisms, biochemical pathways and broader cellular function. Conventional strategies for expression profiling such as Northern blot, Reverse northern blot, Reverse transcriptase-polymerase chain reaction (RT-PCR), Nuclease protection, Enzyme-linked immunosorbent assay (ELISA), Western blot, *in situ* hybridization and immunohistochemistry are optimized for single gene analysis. Although it is possible to modify at least some of these techniques for multiplexing, the procedure becomes increasingly technically cumbersome. For genome wide expression analysis it is necessary to develop technologies that have a high degree of automation since in any living organism thousands of genes and their products function in a complicated and orchestrated way. DNA microarrays were developed in response to the need for a high-throughput, efficient and comprehensive strategy that can simultaneously measure all the genes, or a large defined subset, encoded by a genome[421,422]. Several different methodologies including differential display PCR, northern blots, quantitative PCR, serial analysis of gene expression (SAGE)[423,424] and TIGR Orthologous Gene Alignments (TOGA)[425,426] are used alongside microarrays as research tools.

With an initial focus in the post genomic era on tracking gene expression changes for target identification, microarray applications soon widened to span the entire drug discovery pipeline[427,428,429,430]. DNA microarrays are

---

[421] Schena, M., Shalon, D., Davis, R.W., Brown, P.O., 1995. Quantitative monitoring of gene expression patterns with a complementary DNA microarray. Science 270,467-470.

[422] Schena, M., Shalon, D., Heller, R., Chai, A., Brown, P.O., Davis, R.W., 1996. Parallel human genome analysis: microarray-based expression monitoring of 1000 genes. Proceedings of the National Academy of Sciences of the United States of America. 93,10614 –10619.

[423] Yamamoto, M., Wakatsuki, T., Hada, A., Ryo, A., 2001. Use of serial analysis of gene expression (SAGE) technology. Journal of Immunological Methods. 250 (1-2), 45-66.

[424] Bertelsen, A. H., Velculescu, V.E., 1998. High-throughput gene expression analysis using SAGE. Drug Discovery Today. 3(4), 152-159.

[425] Lee,S. M., Li, M. L., Tse, Y. C., Leung, S. C., Lee, M.M., Tsui, S. K., Fung, K. P., Lee, C. Y., Waye, M. M.,2002. Paeoniae Radix, a Chinese herbal extract, inhibit hepatoma cells growth by inducing apoptosis in a p53 independent pathway. Life Sciences 71 (19), 2267-22 77.

[426] Sogayar, M.C., *et. al.,* 2004, Transcript Finishing Initiative: A transcript finishing initiative for closing gaps in the human transcriptome. Genome Research. 14(7), 1413-1423.

[427] Smith, C., 2004. Drug discovery in reverse. Nature. 428(6979), 227.

[428] Debouck, C., Goodfellow, P.N., 1999. DNA microarrays in drug discovery and development. Nature Genetics. 21(1), 48-50.

[429] Gerhold, D.L., Jensen, R.V., Gullans, S.R., 2002. Better therapeutics through microarrays. Nature Genetics. 32, 547-51.

[430] Reynolds, M.A., 2002. Microarray technology GEM microarrays and drug discovery. Journal of Industrial Microbiology and Biotechnology. 28(3), 180-185.

being used to study the transcriptional profile in various physiological and pathological conditions, leading to the mining of novel genes and molecular markers for diagnosis, prediction or prognosis of those specific states[431,432]. Inspired by the success in the DNA microarray field, **protein arrays** were developed to meet the demands of proteomics research[433,434,435]. Protein microarrays are mainly applied to protein function studies, screening the production of antibodies and recombinant proteins[436], discovery of proteins implicated in disease or those that are potential drug targets, rapid detection or diagnosis of disease[437,438], screening for protein-protein, DNA-protein and enzyme-

---

[431] Koppal, T., 2004. Microarrays: Migrating from Discovery to Diagnostics. Drug Discovery and Development. 7(2), 30-34.

[432] Gebauer, M., 2004. Microarray applications: emerging technologies and perspectives. Drug Discovery Today. 9(21), 915-917.

[433] Huang, J.X., Mehrens, D., Wiese, R., Lee, S., Tam, S.W., Daniel, S., Gilmore, J., Shi, M., Lashkari, D., 2001. High-throughput genomic and proteomic analysis using microarray technology. Clinical Chemistry. 47 (10), 1912-1916.

[434] Merchant, M., Weinberger, S.R., 2000. Recent advancements in surface enhanced laser desorption/ionization time-of-flight mass spectrometry. Electrophoresis. 21, 1164-1177.

[435] Zhu, H., Bilgin, M., Bangham, R., Hall, D., Casamayor, A., Bertone, P., Lan, N., Jansen, R., Bidlingmaier, S., Houfek, T., Mitchell, T., Miller, P., Dean, R.A., Gerstein, M., Snyder, M., 2001. Global analysis of protein activities using proteome chips. Science. 293(5537), 2101-2105.

[436] Kersten, B., Feilner, T., Kramer, A., Wehrmeyer, S., Possling, A., Witt, I., Zanor, M.I., Stracke, R., A., Lueking, J., Kreutzberger, H., Lehrach., Cahill, D.J., 2003. Generation of Arabidopsis protein chips for antibody and serum screening. Plant Molecular Biology. 52(5), 999-1010.

[437] Haab, B.B., 2001. Advances in protein microarray technology for protein expression and interaction profiling. Current Opinion in Drug Discovery Development. 4(1), 116-123.

[438] Kumble, K.D., 2003. Protein microarrays: new tools for pharmaceutical development. Analytical and Bioanalytical Chemistry. 377(5), 812-819.

substrate interactions[439,440]. High-density human protein arrays are undermined by the incomplete knowledge of full-length human gene clones and the vast idiosyncrasies of proteins with respect to stability and structure[441]. While protein microarrays may not have reached the stage of maturity of DNA microarrays, recent developments have shown that many of the barriers holding back the technology can be overcome[442,443]. During the past five years, protein and antibody arrays have emerged as powerful tools that complement DNA microarrays. A genome-scale protein microarray has been demonstrated for identifying protein-protein interactions as well as for rapid identification of protein binding to a particular drug[444]. Furthermore, protein microarrays have also been used to measure the absolute concentration of small molecules. Besides their capacity for parallel diagnostics, microarrays can be more sensitive than traditional methods such as enzyme-linked immunosorbent assay, mass spectrometry or high-performance liquid chromatography-based assays.

Recently cell-based arrays employing matrices of living cells engineered to express select proteins have rapidly

---

[439] MacBeath, G., Schreiber, S.L., 2000. Printing proteins as microarrays for high-throughput function determination. Science. 289(5485), 1760-1763.

[440] Templin, M.F., Stoll, D., Schrenk, M., Traub, P.C., Vohringer, C.F., Joos, T.O., 2002. Protein microarray technology. Drug Discovery Today. 7(15), 815-22.

[441] Kodadek, T., 2001. Protein microarrays: prospects and problems. Chemistry and Biology. 8(2), 105-15.

[442] Schweitzer, B., Predki, P., Snyder, M., 2003. Microarrays to characterize protein interactions on a whole-proteome scale. Proteomics. 3(11), 2190-2199.

[443] Lueking, A., Cahill, D.J., Mullner, S., 2005. Protein biochips: A new and versatile platform technology for molecular medicine. Drug Discovery Today. 10(11), 789-794.

[444] Dufva, M., Christensen, C.B. , 2005. Diagnostic and analytical applications of protein microarrays. Expert Rev Proteomics 2(1),41-48.

emerged as versatile tools for the high-throughput analysis of gene function. Protein-protein interactions can be systematically assayed in a pair-wise manner with a defined library of protein partners[445]. Such an approach can facilitate genome-scale studies on different aspects of protein function, including biochemical activities, gene disruption phenotypes, and protein-protein interactions[446]. Another version of living arrays called transfection microarray has been demonstrated as an alternative to protein microarrays for the identification of drug targets, and as an expression cloning system for the discovery of gene products that alter cellular physiology. Reverse-transfection mediated cellular microarrays contain thousands of distinct cell clusters, each of which produces a protein encoded by a specific expression vector. Transfected cell microarrays expressing 192 different cDNAs, were used to identify proteins involved in tyrosine kinase signalling, apoptosis and cell adhesion, and with distinct sub-cellular distributions[27]. An siRNA transfected cell microarray has been developed to facilitate large-scale, high-throughput functional genomics studies using RNAi [447].

Chemical microarrays, which are arrays of small organic compounds, represent a novel approach towards

---

[445] Uetz, P., Giot, L., Cagney, G., Mansfield, T.A., Judson, R.S., Knight, J.R., Lockshon, D., Narayan, V., Srinivasan, M., Pochart, P., Qureshi, E.A., Li, Y., Godwin, B., Conover, D., Kalbfleisch, T., Vijayadamodar, G., Yang, M., Johnston, M., Fields, S., Rothberg, J.M., 2000. A comprehensive analysis of protein–protein interactions in Saccharomyces cerevisiae. Nature. 403, 623-627.

[446] Qureshi, A.E., Cagney, G., 2000. Large-scale functional analysis using peptide or protein arrays. Nature Biotechnology. 18(4), 393-397.

[447] Junaid, Z., David, M.S., 2001. Microarrays of cells expressing defined cDNAs. Nature. 411, 107 – 110.

[448] Mousses, S., Caplen, N.J., Cornelison, R., Weaver, D., Basik, M., Hautaniemi, S., Elkahloun, A.G., Lotufo, R.A., Choudary, A., Dougherty, E.R., Suh, E., Kallioniemi, O., 2003. RNAi microarray analysis in cultured mammalian cells. Genome Research. 13(10), 2341 –2347.

analysis of chemical libraries. They are widely used to analyze the interaction of proteins with organic compounds in a miniaturized and high-throughput fashion[449,450]. Several modified technologies spanning a wide range of macromolecular microarrays to cell arrays have opened new horizons in molecular and physiological systems.

Applications of DNA Microarrays in Herbal Drug Research

A systems biology approach that integrates such large and diverse sources of information will serve to make useful biological predictions about the pharmacological effects of natural products[451]. DNA microarrays provide a suitable high-throughput platform for such an approach and can be a versatile tool in the research and development of drugs from natural products. In natural products, a broad repertoire of chemical entities act together on multiple targets that makes it necessary to study the changes in expression of multiple genes simultaneously. DNA microarrays can be used for analysis of such combinatorial gene control to make useful predictions with respect to their molecular mechanisms of action, target specificity, toxicity etc.

The applications of DNA microarray technology in herbal drug research and development are discussed with

---

[449] Lam, K. S., Manat, R., 2002. From combinatorial chemistry to chemical microarray. Current Opinion in Chemical Biology. 6(3), 353-358.

[450] Dickopf, S., Frank, H. D., Junker, S., Maier, G., Metz, H., Ottleben, H., Rau, N., Schellhaas, K., Schmidt, R., Sekul, C., Vanier, D., Vetter, J., Czech, M., Lorenz, H., Matter, M., Schudok, H., Schreuder, D.W., Will, H.P., Nestler., 2004. Custom chemical microarray production and affinity fingerprinting for the S1 pocket of factor VIIa. Analytical Biochemistry. 335(1): 50-7.

[451] Wagner, H., 1999. New approaches in phytopharmacological research. Pure Appl. Chem. 71,1649-1654.

suitable examples. Important applications include[452,453,454,455]: First, in Pharmacodynamics, the main applications are for the discovery of new diagnostic and prognostic indicators and biomarkers of therapeutic response; elucidation of molecular mechanism of action of an herb, its formulations or its phytochemical components and identification and validation of new molecular targets for herbal drug development. Second, in Pharmacogenomics, the main uses are for the prediction of potential side-effects of the herbal drug during preclinical activity and safety studies; identification of genes involved in conferring drug sensitivity or resistance and prediction of patients most likely to benefit from the drug and use in general pharmacogenomic studies. Thirdly, in Pharmacognosy, the applications are for correct botanical identification and authentication of crude plant materials as part of standardization and quality control. These applications are described here with some examples.

DNA Microarrays in Pharmacodynamics

Herbal products are usually whole herbs, whose formulations or extracts consist of several bioactive compounds. With the increased demand for scientifically validated and standardized herbal products there is a need for better understanding of the molecular mechanisms underlying their biological activity. Although the physiological actions of many herbal drugs are being studied

---

[452] Clarke, P.A., te Poele, R., Wooster, R., Workman, P., 2001. Gene expression microarray analysis in cancer biology, pharmacology, and drug development: progress and potential. Biochemical Pharmacology. 62(10), 1311-1136.

[453] Butte A., 2002. The use and analysis of microarray data. Nature Reviews in Drug Discovery 1(12), 951-960.

[454] Crowther , D. J., 2002. Applications of microarrays in the pharmaceutical industry. Current Opinion in Pharmacology. 2(5), 551-554.

[455] Klapa, M. I., Quackenbush, J., 2003. The quest for the mechanisms of life. Biotechnology and Bioengineering 84(7), 739-742.

at the molecular level, it remains unclear how individual phytochemical components of herbs contribute to biological activities. Examples of the applications of microarray-based gene expression studies in elucidating molecular mechanisms of action of pure compounds, different phytochemical groups and herbal extracts are discussed here.

Purified Compounds

Modulation of gene expression by *Centella asiatica* triterpenes[456], *Tripterygium hypoglaucum* (levl.) Hutch (Celastraceae) alkaloids[457], and *Anemarrhena asphodeloides* Bunge. saponins[458], were studied with gene microarrays. The identification of genes modulated by these compounds provides the basis for a molecular understanding of the pathways involved in bioactivity, and opportunities for the quantitative correlation of this activity with clinical effectiveness at a molecular level. Similarly, using DNA microarrays it was possible to identify common and distinct genes related to anti-proliferative activities of *Coptidis rhizoma* and its major component berberine in human pancreatic cancer cell lines[459].

---

[456] Coldren, C.D., Hashim, P., Ali, J. M., Oh, S. K., Sinskey A. J., Rha C., 2003. Gene expression changes in the human fibroblast induced by Centella asiatica triterpenoids. Planta Medica 69(8), 725-732.

[457] Zhuang, W. J., Fong, C. C., Cao, J., Ao, L., Leung, C. H., Cheung, H. Y., Xiao, P. G., Fong, W. F., Yang M.S.,2004.Involvement of NF-kappaB and c-myc signaling pathways in the apoptosis of HL-60 cells induced by alkaloids of Tripterygium hypoglaucum (levl.) Hutch. Phytomedicine. 11(4), 295-302.

[458] Li, Z. S., Li, D. L., Huang, J., Ding, Y., Ma, B. P., Wang S. Q., 2003. Investigations on the molecular mechanisms of saponins from Anemarrhena asphodeloides Bunge using oligonucleotide microarrays. Yao Xue Xue Bao. 38(7), 496-500.

[459] Iizuka, N., Oka, M., Yamamoto, K., Tangoku, A., Miyamoto, K., Miyamoto, T., Uchimura, S., Hamamoto Y., Okita K., 2003. Identification of common or distinct genes related to antitumor activities of a medicinal herb and its major component by oligonucleotide microarray. International Journal of Cancer. 107(4), 666-672.

The gene expression pattern of inferior colliculus from DBA/2J mice with audiogenic seizure (AGS) and those treated with Qingyangshenylycosides (QYS), a traditional Chinese medicine, were examined. Gene expression analysis revealed that QYS prevents many of the AGS induced gene expression changes. The data provided important information regarding the molecular mechanisms of AGS and the mechanism of action of QYS[460]. A gene chip, (Rat Genome U34A) was used to elucidate the gene regulatory pattern of Epimedium flavonoids (EF) in immune homeostasis remodeling in the aged rats. The results showed that expression pattern characterized by up-regulation of apoptosis promoting gene expression and down-regulation of apoptosis inhibiting gene expression, is the important gene background of immuno-homeostasis imbalance in the aged. The role of EF is to reverse these abnormal changes of gene expressions to reconstruct a beneficial equilibrium and to further remodel immuno-homeostasis in the aged[461].

The mechanism of herbal glycoside recipes retrieving deficient ability of spatial learning memory in mice suffering from cerebral ischemia/repurfusion was studied using a DNA micoarray system. The gene expression pattern was analyzed in the groups that showed increased ability of spatial learning. A 1.8-fold increase in expression was observed for many genes (38–46) including genes in cell cycle regulation, signal transduction, nerve system transcription factors, DNA binding protein, etc. Nine genes related to retrieving deficient ability of spatial learning

[460] Li, X., Hu, Y., 2005. Gene expression profiling reveals the mechanism of action of anticonvulsant drug QYS. Brain Research Bulletin 66(2), 99-105.

[461] Chen, Y., Shen Z. Y., Chen W. H., 2004. Molecular mechanism of epimedium flavonoids in immune homeostasis remodeling in aged rats revealed by lymphocyte gene expression profile. Zhongguo Zhong Xi Yi Jie He Za Zhi. 24(1), 59-62.

memory treated with glycoside recipes were found in this study[462].

Chronic cocaine use is known to elicit changes in the pattern of gene expression within the brain. The hippocampus plays a critical role in learning and memory and may also play a role in mediating behaviors associated with cocaine abuse. To profile the gene expression response of the hippocampus to chronic cocaine treatment, cDNA hybridization arrays were used to illuminate cocaine-regulated genes in rats treated non-contingently with a binge model of cocaine[463]. Similarly, using DNA microarray analysis, gene expression changes with chronic morphine and antagonist-precipitated withdrawal in two brain regions involved in behavioural effects of morphine in both mice and rats, were characterized[464].

Si-Jun-Zi decoction (SJZD), a traditional Chinese herbal prescription, has been used clinically for treating patients with disorders of the digestive system. Previous studies indicated that the polysaccharides of SJZD are the active components contributing towards its pharmacological effects in improving gastrointestinal function and immunity. SJZD polysaccharide was found to have protective effect and enhanced re-epithelialization on wounded IEC-6 cells. To elucidate the modulatory effect of

---

[462] Wang, Z., Du, Q., Wang, F., Liu, Z., Li, B., Wang A., Wang Y., 2004. Microarray analysis of gene expression on herbal glycoside recipes improving deficient ability of spatial learning memory in ischemic mice. Journal of Neurochemistry. 88(6), 1406

[463] Freeman, W. M. Brebner, K., Lynch, W. J., Robertson, D. J., Roberts, D. C., Vrana, K. E., 2001. Cocaine-responsive gene expression changes in rat hippocampus. Neuroscience. 108(3), 371-380.

[464] McClung, C. A., Nestler, E. J., Zachariou, V., 2005. Regulation of gene expression by chronic morphine and morphine withdrawal in the locus ceruleus and ventral tegmental area. Journal of Neuroscience 25(25), 6005-6015.

polysaccharides of SJZD on wounded IEC-6 cells at the molecular level, an oligonucleotide microarray was employed to study differential gene expression of treated IEC-6 cells and the candidate genes were validated by RT-PCR. There was increased expression of genes coding for ion channels and transporters, which are critical to cell migration and restoration of wounded intestinal cells, suggesting a possible mechanism for re-epithelialization[465].

Extracts

High-density oligonucleotide microarrays have been used for pioneer studies on the multiple gene expression effects exhibited by *Ginkgo biloba* extract EGb 761, changing traditional pharmacology and medicine concepts[466]. *Ginkgo biloba* leaf extract (EGb 761) has been known to have neuroprotective effects ranging from molecular to cellular in animal and human studies, however, the mechanisms remain unclear. DNA microarray based analyses has largely helped in identifying its targets and mechanism of action. High-density oligonucleotide microarrays were used to define the transcriptional effects in the cortex and hippocampus of mice whose diets were supplemented with the herbal extract. This study reveals that diets supplemented with *Ginkgo biloba* extract have notable neuromodulatory effects *in vivo* and illustrates the utility of genome-wide expression monitoring to investigate the

---

[465] Liu, L., Han, L., Wong, D. Y., Yue, P. Y., Ha, W. Y., Hu, Y. H., Wang P. X., Wong R. N., 2005.Effects of Si-Jun-Zi decoction polysaccharides on cell migration and gene expression in wounded rat intestinal epithelial cells. British Journal of Nutrition. 93(1), 21-29.

[466] Christen,Y., Olano-Martin, E., Packer, L.,2002. Egb 761 in the postgenomic era: new tools from molecular biology for the study of complex products such as Ginkgo biloba extract. Cellular and Molecular Biology. 48(6), 593-599.

biological actions of complex extracts[467]. Further, DNA microarray analyses revealed that transcription of multiple apoptosis-related genes is either up- or down-regulated in cells treated with EGb 761. These results suggest that inhibition of apoptotic machinery may, at least in part, mediate multiple neuroprotective effects of EGb 761 [468]. Mechanism of cytostatic action of EGb 761 was elucidated with the help of DNA microarray and the genes important for tumor growth were identified[469].

Ginkgo extract and one of its terpenoid constituents, ginkgolide B, inhibited the proliferation of a highly aggressive human breast cancer cell line and xenografts of this cell line in nude mice. cDNA microarray analyses have shown that exposure of human breast cancer cells to a Ginkgo extract altered the expression of genes that are involved in the regulation of cell proliferation, cell differentiation or apoptosis, and that exposure of human bladder cancer cells to a Ginkgo extract produced an adaptive transcriptional response that augmented antioxidant status and inhibited DNA damage [470].

Water-extract of Paeoniae Radix has an inhibitory effect on the growth of both HepG2 and Hep3B cell lines. Using

---

[467] Watanabe, C. M., Wolffram, S., Ader, P., Rimbach, G., Packer, L., Maguire, J. J., Schultz P.G., Gohil K., 2001. The in vivo neuromodulatory effects of the herbal medicine Ginkgo biloba. Proceedings of the National Academy of Sciences of the United States of America 98(12), 6577-6580.

[468] Smith, J. V., Burdick, A. J., Golik, P., Khan, I., Wallace, D., Luo Y., 2002. Anti-apoptotic properties of Ginkgo biloba extract EGb 761 in differentiated PC12 cells. Cellular and Molecular Biology 48(6), 699-707.

[469] Li, W., Pretner E., Shen, L., Drieu, K., Papadopoulos, V., 2002.Common gene targets of Ginkgo biloba extract (EGb 761) in human tumor cells: relation to cell growth. Cellular and Molecular Biology. 48(6), 655-662.

[470] DeFeudis, F. V., Papadopoulos, V., Drieu, K., 2003. Ginkgo biloba extracts and cancer: a research area in its infancy. Fundamental and Clinical Pharmacology 17(4), 405-417.

cDNA microarray technology and RT-PCR analysis, the drug targets of Paeoniae Radix in inhibition of tumor cells growth were elucidated[471].

Several studies have indicated that extracts of *S. barbata* have growth inhibitory effects on a number of human cancers. However, the mechanism underlying the antitumor activity was unclear. cDNA microarray analysis showed that 16 genes, involved in DNA damage, cell cycle control, nucleic acid binding and protein phosphorylation, underwent more than 5-fold change. This data indicated that these processes are involved in *S. barbata*-mediated killing of cancer cells[472].

The effect of *Syzygium aromaticum* (L.) Merrill and Perry (clove) extract on tissues that regulate glucose metabolism was studied by analysis of gene expression using DNA microarray. The data showed that the extract acts like insulin in hepatocytes and hepatoma cells by reducing phosphoenolpyruvate carboxykinase and glucose 6-phosphatase gene expression. Much like insulin, clove-mediated repression was reversed by PI3K inhibitors and N-acetylcysteine. Moreover, clove and insulin were found to regulate the expression of many of the same genes in a similar manner. These results indicate a potential role for compounds derived from clove as insulin-mimetic agents[473].

---

[471] Lee, Y., Sultana, R., Pertea, G., Cho, J., Karamycheva, S., Tsai, J., Parvizi, B., Cheung, F., Antonescu, V., White, J., Holt, I., Liang, F., Quackenbush, J., 2002. Cross-referencing eukaryotic genomes: TIGR Orthologous Gene Alignments (TOGA). Genome Research. 12(3),493-502

[472] Yin, X. Zhou, J. Jie, C. Xing, D., Zhang, Y., 2004. Anticancer activity and mechanism of Scutellaria barbata extract on human lung cancer cell line A549. Life Sciences 75(18), 2233-2244.

[473] Prasad, R. C. Herzog, B. Boone, B. Sims, L., Waltner-Law, M., 2005. An extract of Syzygium aromaticum represses genes encoding hepatic gluconeogenic enzymes. Journal of Ethnopharmacology 96(1-2), 295-301

A cDNA microarray study demonstrated significant inhibition of inducible endothelial CD36 expression, a novel cardioregulatory gene, by IH636 grape seed proanthocyanidin extract [474].

Both the prototypic tricyclic antidepressant imipramine (IMI) and the extract of St John's wort (SJW) can be effective in the treatment of major depressive disorder. Affymetrix chips were used to study hypothalamic gene expression in rats treated with SJW or IMI to test the hypothesis that chronic antidepressant treatment by various classes of drugs results in shared patterns of gene expression that may underlie their therapeutic effects. SJW treatment differentially regulated 66 genes and expression sequence tags (ESTs) and IMI treatment differentially regulated 74 genes and ESTs. Six common transcripts in response to both treatments were found. Both treatments also affected different genes that are part of the same cell function processes, such as glycolytic pathways and synaptic function. The data support the hypothesis that chronic antidepressant treatment by drugs of various classes may result in a common, final pathway of changes in gene expression in a discrete brain region [475].

DNA Microarray can be used for activity-guided fractionation of herbal extracts in order to determine active principles. The pharmacogenomic activities of *Anoectochilus formosanus* extract as a crude phytocompound mixture

---

[474] Bagchi, D., Sen, C. K., Ray, S. D., Das, D. K., Bagchi, M., Preuss, H. G., Vinson. J. A., 2003. Molecular mechanisms of cardioprotection by a novel grape seed proanthocyanidin extract. Mutation Research. 523-524, 87-97.

[475] Wong, M. L., O'Kirwan, F., Hannestad, J. P., Irizarry, K. J., Elashoff D., Licinio. J., 2004. St John's wort and imipramine-induced gene expression profiles identify cellular functions relevant to antidepressant action and novel pharmacogenetic candidates for the phenotype of antidepressant treatment response. Molecular Psychiatry. 9(3), 237-251.

were compared to those conferred by the single-compound drug, plumbagin in MCF-7 cancer cells. This study offers evidence to support the search for fractionated medicinal herb extracts or phytocompound mixtures, in addition to single-compound drugs, as defined therapeutic agents[476].

DNA Microarrays in Pharmacogenomics

Pharmacogenomics is the study of genes and the gene products (proteins) essential for pharmacological or toxicological responses to pharmaceutical agents. cDNA microarray or oligonucleotide-based DNA chip technology can be a powerful tool to analyze simultaneously the gene expression profiles that are induced or repressed by xenobiotics[477]. DNA microarray techniques might prove to be a reliable basis for predicting the response (or lack of response) of individuals to herbal drugs.

An attempt has been made to develop microarray genotyping system for the multiplex analysis of a panel of single nucleotide polymorphisms (SNPs) in genes encoding proteins involved in blood pressure regulation, and to apply this system in a pilot study demonstrating its feasibility in the pharmacogenetics of an anti-hypertensive drug response[478].

---

[476] Yang, N. S. Shyur, L. F. Chen, C. H., Wang, S. Y., Tzeng, C. M., 2004. Medicinal herb extract and a single-compound drug confer similar complex pharmacogenomic activities in mcf-7 cells. Journal of Biomedical Science 11(3), 418-422.

[477] Rushmore, T. H., Kong, A. N. 2002. Pharmacogenomics, regulation and signaling pathways of phase I and II drug metabolizing enzymes. Current Drug Metabolism 3(5), 481-490.

[478] Liljedahl, U., Karlsson, J., Melhus, H., Kurland, L., Lindersson, M., Kahan, T., Nystrom, F., Lind, L., Syvanen, A. C., 2003. A microarray minisequencing system for pharmacogenetic profiling of antihypertensive drug response. Pharmacogenetics 13(1): 7-17.

Technologies designed to characterize genes and their products on a discovery scale are now having an impact on many areas of biology, including toxicology. Toxicogenomics is the sub-discipline that merges genomics with toxicology. Microarray analysis of gene expression has become a powerful approach for exploring the biological effects of drugs and other chemicals. In toxicology research, gene expression profiling facilitates mechanism-based research on toxicant action by comparing results for an experimental compound with a database. Recently several studies have demonstrated the utility of microarray analysis for studying genome-wide effects of xenobiotics and the rapid identification of toxic hazards for novel drug candidates[479,480].

An example of such a platform is ToxBlot II, a custom microarray containing cDNAs representing 12,564 human genes chosen on the basis of their potential relevance to a broad range of toxicities. ToxBlot II allows the simultaneous expression profiling of genes representing entire cellular pathways, facilitating a very detailed investigation of potential mechanisms of toxicity[481]. Microarray based gene expression profile screens that focus on genes that are relevant to toxicity can be a useful tool for prediction of potential side-effects of herbal drugs during preclinical development and toxicology studies.

---

[479] Amin, R .P., Hamadeh, H.K., Bushel, P.R., Bennett, L., Afshari, C. A., Paules, R.S., 2002.Genomic interrogation of mechanism(s) underlying cellular responses to toxicants. Toxicology 181(0), 555-563.

[480] Waring, J.F., Gum, R., Morfitt, D., Jolly, R. A., Ciurlionis, R., Heindel, M., Gallenberg, L., Buratto, B., Ulrich, R.G., 2002. Identifying toxic mechanisms using DNA microarrays: evidence that an experimental inhibitor of cell adhesion molecule expression signals through the aryl hydrocarbon nuclear receptor. Toxicology 181(0), 537-550.

[481] Pennie, W. D., 2002. Custom cDNA microarrays; technologies and applications. Toxicology 181-182, 551-554.

cDNA microarray analysis was used to study the expression level of genes in oral fibroblast cell lines in response to exposure to ripe areca nut extract. The results showed up-regulation of IL-6 expression and down-regulation of PDGFR, APP-1 and KGF-1 expressions in multiple cell lines assayed. The down-regulation of KGF-1 expression in oral fibroblast cell lines potentially impairs the proliferation of overlying keratinocytes, which could partially explain the frequent epithelial atrophy observed in chronic areca chewers in vivo. This study established a novel toxicogenomic database for areca nut extract[482]. cDNA microarray analysis was also used to analyse the mRNA expression patterns of 1,177 genes in ten oral cancer patients with betel quid chewing history. This study provides pilot data for understanding the pathogenesis of oral cancer in countries like Taiwan where betel quid chewing is prevalent[483].

Recent studies have highlighted that concurrent use of herbs may mimic, magnify, or oppose the effect of drugs[484,485]. These interactions will be of particular importance of herbal products are to be brought to countries where a solid allopathic basis already exists. DNA Microarray can be used for studying herb-drug interactions, and the mechanisms underlying these interactions.

---

[482] Ko, S.Y., Lin, S.C., Chang, K.W., Liu, C.J., Chang, S.S., Lu, S.Y., Liu T.Y., 2003. Modulation of KGF-1 gene expression in oral fibroblasts by ripe areca nut extract. Journal of Oral Pathology and Medicine 32(7), 399-407.

[483] Tsai, W.C., Tsai, S.T., Ko, J.Y., Jin, Y.T., Li,C., Huang, W., Young, K.C., Lai, M.D., Liu, H.S., Wu, L.W., 2004.The mRNA profile of genes in betel quid chewing oral cancer patients. Oral Oncol.40, 418-426.

[484] Fugh-Berman, A., 2000. Herb-drug interactions. Lancet. 355(9198), 134-138.

[485] Coxeter, P. D., McLachlan, A. J., Duke C. C., Roufogalis, B. D., 2004. Herb-drug interactions: an evidence based approach. Current Medicinal Chemistry 11(11), 1513-1525.

Several botanical constituents in PC-SPES, a botanical preparation, inhibit tumor growth through cell cycle arrest and apoptosis. LNCaP prostate carcinoma cells were treated with PC-SPES, and changes in gene expression were determined by complementary DNA (cDNA) microarray hybridization and northern blot analyses. mRNA levels of á-tubulin decreased sevenfold. The results show that PC-SPES may interfere with microtubule polymerization. This activity has implications for the clinical management of patients with advanced prostate cancer who may be taking PC-SPES concurrently with microtubule-modulating chemotherapeutic agents, such as paclitaxel[486].

DNA Microarray in Pharmacognosy

DNA polymorphism-based assays have been developed for the identification of herbal medicines[487,488]. In this approach, small amounts of DNA are amplified by the polymerase chain reaction and the reaction products are analyzed by gel electrophoresis, sequencing, or hybridization with species-specific probes. Recently, microarrays have been applied for the DNA sequence-based identification of medicinal plants[489,490].

---

[486] Bonham, M. J., Galkin, A., Montgomery, B., Stahl, W. L., Agus, D., Nelson, P. S., 2002. Effects of the Herbal Extract PC-SPES on Microtubule Dynamics and Paclitaxel-Mediated Prostate Tumor Growth Inhibition. Journal of the National Cancer Institute 94(21), 1641-1647.

[487] Joshi, K., Chavan, P., Warude, D., Patwardhan, B., 2004. Molecular markers in herbal drug technology. Current Science. 87 (2), 159-65.

[488] Warude, D., Chavan, P., Joshi, K., Patwardhan, B., 2003. Isolation of DNA from fresh and dry samples having highly acidic tissues. Plant Molecular Biology Reporter, 21, 1-6

[489] Carles, M., Lee,T., Moganti, S., Lenigk, R., Tsim, K. W., Ip, N. Y., I Hsing, M., Sucher, N. J., 2002. Chips and Qi: microcomponent-based analysis in traditional Chinese medicine. Fresenius Journal of Analytical Chemistry. 371(2),190-194.

[490] Trau, D., Lee, T. M., Lao, A. I., Lenigk, R., Hsing, I. M., Ip, N.Y. , Carles, M. C., Sucher, N.J., 2002. Genotyping on a complementary metal oxide semiconductor silicon polymerase chain reaction chip with integrated DNA microarray. Analytical Chemistry 74(13), 3168-3173.

To utilize DNA microarrays for identification and authentication of herbal material, it is necessary to identify a distinct DNA sequence that is unique to each species of medicinal plant. The DNA sequence information is then used to synthesize a corresponding probe on a silicon-based gene chip. These probes are capable of detecting complementary target DNA sequences if present in the test sample being analyzed.

Oligonucleotide probes specific for polymorphisms in the D2 and D3 regions of 26S rDNA gene of several *Fritillaria* species were designed and printed on poly-lysine coated slides to prepare a DNA chip. Differentiation of the various *Fritillaria* species was accomplished based on hybridization of fluorescently labeled PCR products with the DNA chip. The results demonstrated the reliability of using DNA chips to identify different species of *Fritillaria,* and that the DNA chip technology can provide a rapid, high throughput tool for genotyping and plant species authentication[491].

Similarly, using fluorescence-labeled ITS2 sequences as probes, distinctive signals were obtained for the five medicinal *Dendrobium* species listed in the Chinese Pharmacopoeia. The established microarray was able to detect the presence of *D. nobile* in a Chinese medicinal formulation containing nine herbal components[492].

A silicon-based DNA microarray using species-specific oligonucleotide probes is designed and fabricated to identify multiple toxic traditional Chinese medicinal plant species

---

[491] Tsoi, P.Y., Wu, H. S., Wong, M.S., Chen, S. L., Fong, W. F., Xiao, P. G., Yang, M. S., 2003. Genotyping and species identification of Fritillaria by DNA chip technology. Acta Pharmaceutica Sinica. 4, 185-190.

[492] Zhang, Y.B., Wang, J., Wang, Z.T., But P. P., Shaw, P.C., 2003. DNA microarray for identification of the herb of dendrobium species from Chinese medicinal formulations. Planta Medica 69(12), 1172-1174.

by parallel genotyping[493]. Chip-based authentication of medicinal plants may be useful as economical, precise tool for quality control and safety monitoring of herbal pharmaceuticals and neutraceuticals.

Identification of herbal materials, which commonly consist of dried or processed parts, is difficult. This is particularly true for similar looking herbal materials that can often vary greatly in their medicinal properties and market value. DNA microarray based technology can provide an efficient, accurate and cheaper means of testing the authenticity of hundreds of samples simultaneously while conventional chemical methodologies usually take several days for verification. Chip-based authentication of medicinal plants can be useful as a tool for quality control and safety monitoring of herbal pharmaceuticals and neutraceuticals and will significantly add to the medical potential and commercial profitability of herbal products. This application of DNA microarrays will not only benefit the herbal drug industry but also provide a technology platform that can facilitate the identification of herbal products by regulatory authorities.

❏❏❏

---

[493] Carles, M., Cheung, M.K., Moganti, S., Dong, T.T., Tsim, K.W., Ip, N.Y., Sucher, N.J., 2005. A DNA microarray for the authentication of toxic traditional Chinese medicinal plants. Planta Medica 71(6), 580-584.

14 Pharmacogenomics and Ethnopharmacology

Genetics forms the basis of human life. All individuals have a physical and physiological self, determined by the interactions of genes and environment. Pharmacogenetics is the connotation used to study how heritability affects an individual's response to drugs.[494] The term 'Pharmacogenomics' represents systematic identification of all human genes, their products, interindividual variation and intraindividual variation in expression and function over time. It focuses on candidate genes and may include transcriptome and proteome information that affect drug metabolism, pharmacokinetics, and pharmacodynamics. It helps in predicting the patient's response to a drug and to design new drugs[495]. Pharmacogenetics is study of single genes and the effects on drug response while pharmacogenomics is related to overall variation in genome. A gene is considered polymorphic when a mutation appears in more than 1% population, which may be present in the form of single nucleotide polymorphism (SNP), simple sequence length

---

[494] Roses A. Pharmacogenetcs and the practice of medicine. Nature; vol 405; 15 June 2000.

[495] Majid Y. Moridani, The significance of pharmacogenomics in pharmacy education and practice. Am. J. Pharma. Edu. 2005; 69: Article 37.

polymorphism (SSLP) and nucleotide addition or deletion. After the Human Genome Project, study in this field is accelerated dramatically. It was found that out of 1.4 million SNPs identified in the human genome, over 60,000 are present in the coding region[496]. These SNPs lead to miscoding of the various proteins that plays crucial role in the biological processes. If a point mutation is present in the gene coding region for various drug-metabolizing enzymes, drug target and drug transporters, it can lead to many non-therapeutic and unpredictable drug responses. In United States, over two million people suffer from severe adverse drug reactions per year and about 100,000 cases are life threatening[497].

Pharmacogenetics studies accelerated after the 1950's when researchers realized that adverse reactions of drugs could be a consequence of genetic variations in enzyme activity[1]. The observation that the hydrolysis of the muscle relaxant succinylcholine by butyrylcholinesterase (Phase I reaction) was inherited provided initial stimulus for the study of pharmacogenetics. The subjects who were homozygous for the gene encoding an atypical form of butyrylcholinesterase had altered ability to hydrolyse succinylcholine, thus prolonging the drug induced muscle paralysis and consequent apnea[498]. Approximately 1 in 3500 white subjects were homozygous for this gene[499]. Around the same time, genetic variation in a phase II enzyme N –

---

[496] Evans W. and Howard L. McLeod. Pharmacogenomics — Drug disposition, drug targets, and side effects. N. Engl. J. Med. 2003; 6:538-549

[497] Shastry S. Pharmacogenetics and the concept of individualized medicine. Pharmacogemomics J.2006;6:16-21

[498] Idem. The relation between dose of succinylcholine and duration of apnea in man. J Pharmacol Exp Ther; 1957; 120; 203 – 214.

[499] Kalow W, Gunn DR. Some statistical data on atypical cholinesterase of human serum. Ann Hum Genet; 1959; 23; 239 – 50.

acetyltransferase 2 (NAT 2) was suspected. The drugs metabolized by NAT 2 included the antituberculosis drug isoniazid, antihypertensive hydralazine and antiarrhythmic procainamide. Genetic variation resulted in striking differences in the half life and plasma concentrations of drugs due to fast or slow rates of acetylation.

Genetic polymorphism results in variants of functional importance, which further results in an inactive enzyme, reduced catalytic activity or perhaps even gene duplication. These polymorphisms precipitate into four phenotypic subpopulations of drug metabolizers. Poor metabolizers retain drug in the body for a longer time than normal and hence the plasma concentration of the drug is high for longer period. Intermediate metabolizers retain drug in the body for the optimal period. Extensive metabolizers retain drug in the body for less time and the plasma concentration of the drug is high but for shorter period. Ultra rapid metabolizers metabolize drug much faster and more extensively than all other subpopulations.

Factors Affecting Variability in Drug Response

Individuals show variability in drug responses and disease susceptibility. As a result of inter-individual variation, some patients develop adverse drug reaction while other patients respond positively to the same drug administered at the same dose. This variability often is an outcome of differences in the extent of drug metabolism and, as a result, the drug's rate of elimination. This has a known influence in clinical medicine and also in the development of new drugs. There are number of factors associated that determine drug metabolism[500].

---

[500] Meyer UA. Pharmacogenetics and adverse drug reactions. The Lancet; vol. 356; November 11, 2000.

Factors Affecting Drug Metabolism[501]

Genetic variation: Advances in molecular biology have identified allelic variants of drug metabolizing enzymes (DMEs) with different catalytic activities from those of wild type. The differences involve a variety of molecular mechanisms that lead to a complete lack of catalytic activity, reduction of catalytic activity or enhanced activity in case of gene duplication. These molecular mechanisms result in subpopulations with varied drug metabolizing abilities. A number of genetic polymorphisms are present in several DME genes that lead to altered drug metabolizing abilities.

Environmental: Drug metabolism is modulated by exposure to certain exogenous compounds like concomitantly administered drug (drug-drug interaction), dietary micronutrients, etc. There are two forms of modulation. The first is induction or upregulation of drug metabolism, which occurs by enhanced gene transcription following prolonged exposure to an inducing agent This results in an increase in the rate of metabolism, a decrease in bioavailability and a decrease in the plasma concentration of a drug. e.g. Cigarette smoke produces marked induction of the CYP1A subfamily of enzymes. Secondly, inhibition or down regulation of drug metabolism occurs due to competition in two or more substrates for same active site of the same enzyme determined by relative concentration of substrates and their affinities for the enzyme. This results in an increase in plasma concentration of the drug, and a reduction in metabolism that may further result in drug-induced toxicity such as the CYP450 isoform that is required in the metabolism of many drugs.

Disease factors: The liver is a major organ involved in drug metabolism. Diseases like hepatitis, alcoholic liver

---

[501] Goodman & Gilman's The Pharmacological Basis of Therapeutics; 10th Edition. McGraw Hill.pg 15.

disease, biliary cirrhosis and hepatocarcinomas hamper drug-metabolizing ability of liver. Severity of liver damage is directly proportional to decreases in the rate of drug metabolism. Phase I enzymes like CYP-450 are affected more than phase II enzymes. Other diseases like severe cardiac failure and shock result in decreased perfusion of the liver and impaired metabolism.

Age and sex: Few generalizations are possible regarding clinical importance of age related changes in drug metabolism in an individual patient. Newborn and infants metabolize drugs efficiently but at slower rate than adults. Full maturity occurs after 10 years of age. Many examples indicate differences in drug responsiveness of men and women for certain drugs such as drug metabolizing activity of CYP3A.

Genetic Variability Influencing Drug Response: Genetic and environmental factors interact with each other, which results in variation. Genetic variations are inherited differences. There are a variety of conditions under which the genetic backdrop of an individual will affect their ability to metabolize a drug.

According to the basic principles of pharmacology, a drug molecule must exert some chemical influence on one or more constituents of target cells to produce a pharmacological response. The drug molecules thus need to reach the target cells. Once a drug is administered to the patient, it is first absorbed by the body, and then distributed to the site of its action where it interacts with the target cell[502,5]. Regulatory proteins commonly involved in a drug response include: Drug metabolizing enzymes; Transport proteins; Drug receptors; Enzymes in the pathway of drug action and drug metabolic pathway.

[502] Weinshilboum R. Inheritance and Drug Response. N Engl J Med 2003; 6:348.

Drug Metabolizing Enzymes: There are over thirty families of drug metabolizing enzymes (DMEs) in human beings and which all have genetic variants. Variants may result in functional changes in encoded proteins that consequently affect the metabolism of drugs in the human body[3]. Drug elimination is an irreversible loss of drug from the body and occurs by processes of metabolism and excretion. Most drugs are excreted through urine, either unchanged or as polar metabolites. However, the kidney does not eliminate lipophilic substances efficiently. Most lipophilic drugs are metabolized to more polar products, which are then excreted in urine. Drug metabolism occurs predominantly in the liver, mainly by the enzyme cytochrome P450 system.

Phase I DMEs include Cytochrome P450 enzymes. Enzymes of this family metabolize number of chemically diverse, endogenous and exogenous compounds, including drugs, environmental chemicals, and other xenobiotics. They function as the terminal oxidase in a multicomponent Electron Transport Chain that introduces a single atom of molecular oxygen into the substrate with the other atom being incorporated into water. Cytochrome P450 (CYP450) catalyzes reactions involving hydroxylation, dealkylation, oxidation, sulfoxidation, deamination, dehalogenation and desulfuration[503].

Approximately, 1000 CYP450 enzymes are currently known. Out of these around 50 are functionally active in human beings. These are categorized into 17 families and many sub-families based on the amino acid sequence similarities of the predicted proteins. The term CYP is used for identification of these enzymes.

---

[503] Goodman & Gilman's The Pharmacological Basis of Therapeutics; 10th Edition. McGraw Hill.pg17.

Sequences that are more than 40% identical form same family, identified by an Arabic number. Within a family, sequences with greater than 55% homology are in the same subfamily, identified by a letter; and an Arabic number identifies different isoforms within the subfamily. About 8 to 10 isoforms in the CYP1, CYP2 and CYP3 families are involved in the majority of drug metabolism reactions in human beings. Each individual CYP isoform has a characteristic substrate specificity based on structural features of the substrate. Two or more CYP isoforms and drug metabolizing enzymes are often involved in drug metabolism, leading to formation of many primary and secondary metabolites.

Genetic variation has been seen in the CYP450 enzymes. The following are few examples: CYP2D6: This is the most extensively studied and characterized example of pharmacogenetic variation in drug metabolizing enzyme. The drugs that are metabolized by this enzyme are tricyclic antidepressants, debrisoquine, codeine, clozapine and metoprolol[504]. The allelic variants of CYP2D6 have different drug metabolism phenotypes - poor metabolizers (PM), extensive metabolizers (EM), ultra extensive metabolizers (UEM)[505]. The variants range from single nucleotide polymorphisms (SNPs) that alter the amino acid sequence of the encoded protein to SNPs that altered RNA splicing or deletion of the CYP2D6[3]. The frequently studied alleles are *3, *4, *5 and *10, which are responsible for reduced or null activity of the enzyme.

---

[504] Weinshilboum R. Inheritance and Drug Response. N ENGL J MED 348;6: 529-537.

[505] Adithan C, Gerard N, Naveen AT, Koumaravelou K, Shashindran CH, Krishnamoorthy R. Genotype and allele frequency of CYP2D6 in Tamilian population. Eur J Clin Pharmacol (2003) 59: 517-520.

In Caucasians, the frequencies of allele *4 is 19.5% and in Japanese it is 0% while the frequency of allele *10 in Caucasians is only 2% and that in Japanese it is 38.6%. The frequency of *5 allele in Caucasians and Japanese is 4.1% and 6.2% respectively[3]. In the Indian mainland, these studies were carried out in Tamil Nadu, Kerala and North India. In the Tamilian population the frequency of *3 is 0%, * 4 is 6.6%, *10 is 20.3% and *5 is 0.9%[4].

CYP2C9: This gene is important in the metabolism of drugs like phenytoin, warfarin, tolbutamide, glipizide, losartan and acenocoumarol. There are 12 variant alleles consequent to SNP. Three alleles *1, *2, *3 are frequently identified in all ethnic populations. It has been reported that *2 and *3 have significantly reduced enzyme activity which results in poor metabolism of a drug and possibly to drug toxicity[506]. In a study that was carried out in an Italian population, it was revealed that there were homozygous EM (53.3%), heterozygous EM(35%), UM (8.3%) and PM (3.4%)[507]. In India such study has been carried out in the South and the North India. In a South Indian population there was no significant heterogeneity in the allele frequencies amongst the four south Indian states. The frequencies are *1- 8.8%, *2- 0.4% and *3- 0.8%[508].

CYP3A4: P-450 3A subfamily is predominant isoform in human liver and it contains three known members 3A4,

---

[506] Adithan C, Gerard N, Vasu S, Balakrishnan R, Shashindran CH, Krishnamoorthy R. Allele and genotype frequency of CYP2C9 in Tamil Nadu population. Eur J Clin Pharmacol (2003) 59: 707-709.

[507] Scordo MG, Caputi AP, D'Arrigo C, Fava G, Spina E. Allele and genotype frequencies of CYP2C9, CYP2C19 and CYP2D6 in an Italian population. Pharmacological Research 50 (2004) 195-200.

[508] Jose R, Adithan C, Soya SS *et. al.*, CYP2C9 and CYP2C19 genetic polymorphisms: frequencies in the south Indian population. Blackwell Publishing Fundamental & Clinical Pharmacology (2005);1-5.

3A5 and 3A7. CYP3A4 is abundantly present in human liver and small intestine. The drugs metabolized include nifedipine, cyclosporine, erythromycin, midazolam, alprazolam and triazolam. High interindividual variation is observed in CYP3A4 gene. There are four identified allelic variants. The first frequently observed is CYP3A4*1B. Its frequency was low in white and Hispanic subjects (3.6% - 11%), absent in Chinese and Japanese subjects and much higher in black subjects (53% - 69%). Second allelic variant is CYP3A4*2. This allele has a low frequency in white subjects (2.7%) and was not observed in black or Chinese groups[16].

CYP2C19: This enzyme plays a major role in the metabolism of some clinically important drugs such as omeprazole, diazepam and proguanil. Genetic polymorphism of CYP2C19 occurs with the frequency of 18% to 23% in Japanese subjects, 2% to 5% in white subjects, 11% to 20% in Chinese and 12% in Koreans.[509] The most frequently identified alleles are CYP2C19*2 and *3. The resultant phenotype is poor metabolizers[510].

Phase II DMEs include: Glutathione S-transferases (GSTs): GSTs catalyze conjugation reactions in the phase II of drug metabolism. The anticancer agents are substrates for this enzyme. Glutathione is conjugated with several medications and their oxidative damaging metabolites, but due to conjugation they are generally inactivated.[1] GSTs are also termed as 'a triple threat in detoxification' as they protect cells in either of following ways: a) by enzymatically conjugating eletrophilic reactive xenobiotics; b) by binding

---

[509] Lamba JK, Dhiman RK, Kohli KK. CYP2C19 genetic mutations in North Indians. Clinical Pharmacology & Therapeutics; Volume 68; Number 3; pp. 328-335.

[510] Adithan C, Gerard N, Vasu S, Rosemary J, Shashindran CH, Krishnamoorthy R. Allele and genotype frequency of CYP2C19 in a Tamilian population. Br J Clin Pharmacol 56; 331-333.

reactive substrates and preventing damage to important cellular components; c) by suicide inactivation of enzyme and substrate[511]. GST genes are highly polymorphic and, particularly GSTM1 and GSTT1. Studies have shown that 25% of most populations have complete deletion of GSTM1 and GSTT1[1, 2]. Studies have been carried out to investigate distribution of individuals lacking these enzymes due to homozygous gene deletions. In South India 30.4% lacked the GSTM1 gene while 16.8% lacked GSTT1 and 4.6% lacked both. The frequency of absence GSTM1 is much higher in Caucasians (53.5%) and Japanese (51.3%). Frequency of GSTT1 null genotypes is lower in South Indians than in Japanese (54%) and Afro-Americans (24.1%)[11].

Thiopurine methyltransferase (TPMT): TPMT catalyzes methylation of drug in phase II of the drug metabolism. The drugs related are azathioprine, mercaptopurine and thioguanine are thiopurine agents commonly used for a range of medical indications like leukemia, rheumatic diseases, and inflammatory bowel disease. These thiopurines are inactive prodrugs that require metabolism to thioguanine nucleotides (TGN). The TGN incorporates into DNA to exert cytotoxicity. TPMT inactivates these agents. TPMT activity is highly variable and eight variant alleles have been identified. Three alleles *2, *3A, *3C account for about 95% of intermediate or low enzyme activity; *3A is most common variant (3.2% to 5.7%) in the white population. In Asians, the predominant variant is *3C. The patients with homozygous mutant compound heterozygous genotype are at higher risk of developing severe haematopoietic toxicity if treated with conventional doses of thiopurines.

---

[511] Naveen AT, Adithan C, Padmaja N et al. Glutathione S-transferase M1 and T1 null genotype distribution in South Indians. Eur J Clin Pharmacol (2004) 60: 403-406.

Uridine diphosphate glucuronosyl transferases (UGTs): Glucuronicais is the conjugation reaction wherein UGTs catalyze the transfer of glucuronicacid to aromatic and aliphatic alcohols, carboxylic acids, amines and free sulphahydryl groups to form O-, N-, S- glucuronides respectively[512]. These reactions are responsible for eliminaton of a diverse range of xenobiotics and endogenous compounds. There are 16 functional human UGT genes out of which 6 genes have shown genetic polymorphism: UGT1A1, 1A6, 1A7, 2B4, 2B7, 2B15[513]. UGT1A1 is responsible for the glucuronidation of bilirudin. There are three forms of inheritable unconjugated hyperbilirubinemia: Crigler-Najjar syndrome Type I and II and Gilbert syndrome. Studies have shown that Gilbert syndrome arises from polymorphism in UGT1A1 promoter region containing TA repeat element. The frequency of promoters with decreased activity was found to be highest in African populations and lowest in Asian populations[514]. Studies have been done to show an association between the genetic polymorphisms of the UGT1A7 gene and irinotecan toxicity in cancer patients. One such study in Japan has shown that amongst 26 patients with severe toxicity, allele frequency for UGT1A7*1 was 61.5% while in 92 patients without severe toxicity it was 63.6%, suggesting that determination of UGT1A7 genotypes would not be useful for predicting severe toxicity of irinotecan[515].

---

[512] Rang HP, Dale MM, Ritter JM. Pharmacology; 4th edition. ChurchillLivingstone, Edinburgh.pp: 78-79.

[513] Miners JO, McKinnon RA, Mackenzie PI. Genetic polymorphisms of UDP-glucuronosyltransferases and their functional significance. Toxicology 181-182 (2002); 453-456.

[514] Beutler E, Gelbart T, Demina A. Racial variability in the UDP-glucuronosyltransferase 1 (UGT1A1) promoter: a balanced polymorphism for regulation of bilirubin metabolism? Proc. Natl .Acad. Sci.USA Vol. 95:pp.8170-8174:July 1998. Genetics.

[515] Ando M, Ando Y, Sekido Y, Ando M, Shimokata K, Hasegava Y. Genetic Polymorphisms of the UDP-Glucuronosyltransferase 1A7 Gene and Irinotecan Toxicity in Japanse Cancer Patients. Jpn. J. Cancer Res. 93; 591-597; May 2002.

Drug transporters: Membrane transport proteins are important and involved in absorption of drugs into the intestinal tract, brain and several other tissues. These proteins are also involved in distribution and excretion of drugs. Amongst various ATP-binding proteins, the ATP binding cassette family is one of the most studied. P-glycoprotein is a member of this family that is encoded by the ABCB1 (MDR1) gene. This protein acts as an efflux pump, which exports various substrates, like bilirubin, anticancer agents, immunosuppressive agents, human immunodeficiency virus (HIV) type I protease inhibitor and others outside the cell. Association studies between ABCB1 gene variants and treatment outcome in HIV infected patients receiving combined antiretroviral therapy are being carried out. ABCB1 3435C→T single nucleotide polymorphism (SNP) has shown association with significant differences in plasma concentration of nelfinavir and efavirenz. Patients with the TT genotype showed greater and more rapid recovery of CD4 cell count than patients with CC or CT genotype. SNP in exon 26 (3435C→T) shows considerable ethnic differences in the frequencies of allelic variants. The TT genotype accounts for 0% - 6% of black Africans and African Americans, 20% - 47% of Asians and 24% - 36% of white population.

Drug receptors: Drug interacts with membrane receptors to exert a pharmacological effect. Genetic variations in such drug targets may alter a drug response. Gene polymorphism in various targets such as β2 adrenoreceptor and response to β2 agonist, angiotensin converting enzyme and renoprotective effects of ACE inhibitor, apolipoprotein E and response to HMG co-reductase inhibitors and various others have been studied. β2 adrenoreceptor plays an important role in regulating cardiac, vascular, pulmonary and metabolic functions. β2 adrenoreceptor coded by the ADRB2 gene is extensively investigated for genetic polymorphisms and their clinical importance. SNP resulting in a Arg to Gly amino acid change at codon 16 and a Gln to Glu change at codon 27 are comparatively common. Patients homozygous for Arg16 showed nearly complete desensitization to continuous infusion of isoproterenol with decreasing venodilatation. Patients homozygous for Gly16 had no significant change in venodilatation, regardless of their codon 27 sequence. Patients homozygous for Glu27 showed maximal venodilatation in response to isoproterenol as compared to the homozygous Gln27 genotype, regardless of their codon 16 sequence.

Enzymes variability in Drug pathway/Drug metabolic pathway: Apart from the drug targets on which the drug directly act there are several other targets on which the drug exerts its action indirectly. Mutation in these targets also leads to many complications of drug efficacy and toxicity. Methotrexate is now widely accepted for the treatment of Rheumatoid Arthritis and in various forms of Cancers. Methotrexate enters the cell through an active transport mechanism. Intracellularly, methotrexate is converted to polyglutamate form by the enzyme Folylpolyglutamyl Synthase. The enzyme Gamma Glutamyle Hydrolase can reverse this process. This polyglutamate form of the drug directly inhibits Dihydrofolate Reductase, which reduces dihydrofolate to tetrahydrofolate. Polyglutamate, and hence Methotrexate also inhibit other folate dependent enzyme, Thymidylate Synthase (TYMS), Methylenetetrahydrofolate Reductase and others.

Ethnicity: In order to use genomic knowledge to develop drug and to improve health, we need to know the effect of ethnic differences in different populations. Significant nter-ethnic differences exist polymorphisms of gene encoding drug metabolizing enzymes, transporter and disease associated proteins. Genetic differences are greater within socially defined racial groups than between groups. Additionally, it has been found that genetic diversity decreases in noncoding regions whereas diversity of coding nonsynonymous SNPs is lower in regions containing a known protein sequence motif in individuals of European origin[516].

Drug treatment may be personalized for greater effect if an important genetic variation exists between racial and ethnic groups. By knowing these variants, patients can be classified into low, intermediate and high dose groups. For example, Warfarin therapy shows a wide variation among patients of different ethnicities. This variation could be due to polymorphism in gene encoding vitamin K epoxide reductase complex 1. Accordingly Chinese patients require lower dosage of heparin and Warfarin than Caucasian patients[517]. This is due to biological differences between the two racial groups. Thus, an understanding of the genetic variation between different ethnicities is useful and pharmacogenetics is a major tool for elucidating genetic variability.

Human Genome Project

The genome is the complete DNA of an organism. The human genome is the total DNA content in human cells. Out of the total genome only 2% codes for protein while the rest all is noncoding. In humans, the genome comprises 25 different DNA molecules, a single mitochondrial DNA

---

[516] Freudenberg-Hua Y, Freudenberg J, Winantea J ,Kluck N, Cichon S,Bruss M, Systematic investigation of genetic variability in 111 human gene –implication for studying variable drug response. Pharmacogenomics J. 2005;5:183-192

[517] Yu C., Chan TYK., Critchley J., Woo K.Factors determining the maintenance dose of Warfarin in Chinese patients . Q J Med. 1996;89:127-135

and 24 different nuclear DNA molecules. The amount of DNA within the nucleus is so large that the term genome is often used to mean the set of nuclear DNA. In year 1956, the first physical map of the human genome was determined. Since the 1950's, genetists have had rough idea about the physical map of human genome. A physical map provides information on the linear structure of DNA molecules. To truly understand how the human body functions, it was necessary to obtain a human genetic map. Earlier, classical genetic maps were constructed of drosophila and mouse to determine whether the two gene loci are linked or not. Constructing a classical genetic map was not possible as the frequency of mating between individuals suffering from different genetic disorders is very small. This problem was resolved in late 1970s after the measurement of DNA variation by restriction fragment length polymorphism (RFLPs) method. In 1977, Sanger and his colleagues published their dideoxy DNA sequencing method and four years later they published complete sequence of human mitochondrial DNA.

In 1987, the U.S. Department of Energy Report on Human Genome Initative launched the Human Genome Project (HGP) to understand the variation in DNA among individuals, for which it was necessary to sequence and analyze the genome. The Human Genome Project was formally coordinated by the U.S. Department of Energy and the National Institutes of Health. The HGP attempted to map and sequence 3 billion nucleotides to identify all the the genes contained in the human genome. The project originally was planned for 15 years, but due to advances in technologies it was completed by 2003. The main goals of the HGP include to *identify* all the approximately 20,000-25,000 genes in human DNA; to *determine* the sequences of the 3 billion chemical base pairs that make up human DNA; to *store* this information in databases; to *improve* tools for data analysis; to *transfer* related technologies to the private sector; to *address* the ethical, legal, and social issues that may arise from the project[518].

Before the human genome had been sequenced, the prediction for the total number of human genes was in range of 60,000-100,000 genes. Now, it is believed to have only 30,000-35,000 genes. This draft of the human genome was a major step in understanding phenotypes and the draft sequence is useful to understand which genes are associated with disease. A number of genes have associations with diseases such as breast cancer, muscle disease, cardiovascular disease, diabetes, and arthritis. An understanding of these interactions is developing through the use of human variation maps (SNPs) generated in cooperation with the private sector. These genes and SNPs provide focused targets for the development of effective new therapies[519].

Ayu Genomics

It is possible to examine the Ayurvedic concept of *Prakruti* from a human genome perspective. Permutations and combinations of influencing factors including 111 of Vata, 86 of Pitta and 92 of Kapha give near 800,000 variables. Considering other variable factors like desha (habitat), kala (time), etc. takes this number to over 3,000,000. By applying Dhatu Sarata and the 20 Guna this number tends to infinity. This is how Ayurveda describes the basis of individual variation. The concept of *Prakriti*

---

[518] The U.S. National Human Genome Research Institute (NHGRI) at http://www.nhgri.nih.gov/, The U.S. National Center for Biotechnology Information (NCBI) at http://www.ncbi.nlm.nih.gov/l The nature Genome Gateway at http://www.nature.com/genomics/

[519] Strachan and Read, Human Molecular Genetics.3rd edition, Garland publications (Taylor and FrancisGroup) 2004, New York.

has central role in understanding health and disease in Ayurveda, which is very similar to pharmacogenetics that is expected to become basis of designer medicine[520]. Designer medicine is a pharmaceutical product that will give maximum therapeutic efficacy and high safety to the particular person with particular disorder. The fundamental principles of Ayurvedic system of medicine can be used for creating Designer Medicines. One of the steps towards this is identifying the genetic basis of 'Prakriti' classification if any exists.

Integration of Ayurveda and Genomics[521]

A better understanding of the human genome has helped in understanding the scientific basis of individual variation. If not for the great variability among individuals, medicine might as well be a science and not an art.

After Human Genome Project, Sir Wilam Osler would have changed his view of medicine as an art and not science[522]. While medical practice will continue to remain an art, medicine per se has become science. It has become more predictive, individual and customized. For years physicians have noted individual differences but had no way to predict them. Pharmacogenetics is the study of the hereditary basis for differences in populations' response to a drug. The same dose of a drug will result in elevated plasma concentrations for some patients and low concentrations for others. Some patients will respond well to the drugs, while others will not. A drug might show adverse effects in some patients but not in others. An

---

520 Patwardhan Bhushan, Ayurveda: The Designer Medicine, Indian Drugs, 2000; 37(5), 213-227.

521 Patwardhan Bhushan, Ashok D. B. Vaidya and Mukund Chorghade. (2004) Ayurvedaa and Natural Product Drug Discovery. Current Science, 86 (6), 789-799.

522 Roses Allen, Pharmacogenetics: A Review. Nature 15 June 2000.

example of this is Phenylthiourea related taste blindness, which demonstrated that a chemical sensitivity could be heritable and that chemical sensitivity could serve as a means of distinguishing between individuals. African Blacks had an incidence of around six percent, American Blacks 2-23%, American Whites 30%, Chinese 6% and Eastern Eskimos 40%. All earlier studies indicated that the differences in response to disease and drugs not only differs among populations but is truly individual. The human race is believed to have originated in Africa and has 98% of the genetic make up similar to chimps. Generally speaking, humans are classified into three major groups: The Negroid, Mongoloid, and Caucasoid, who are genetically 99.9% identical. The difference in terms of color, physic, behavior and such is due to single nucleotide polymorphism or SNPs and it just constitutes 1%.

Importance of such individual variations in health and disease is an important basic principle of Ayurveda and was underlined by Charaka 4000 years ago as 'Every individual is different from another and hence should be considered as a different entity.

As many variations are there in the Universe, all are seen in Human being'. AyuGenomics describes the basis of individual variation and it has clear similarities with the pharmacogenomics that is expected to become the basis of designer medicine[12]. Understanding the possible relationship between Prakriti and the human genome will be important. Functionally this will involve creation of three organized databases that are capable of intelligently communicating with each other to give a customized prescription. These are Human constitution (Genotype), Disease constitution (Phenotype) and Drug constitution. A golden triangle[523] consisting of Ayurveda-Modern

[523] Mashelkar R.A. Chitrakoot Declaration, National Botanical Research Institute Convention, 2003.

medicine - Science will converge to form a real discovery engine that can result in newer, safer, cheaper and more effective therapies. It will be in the interest of pharmaceutical companies, researchers and ultimately the global community to respect the traditions and build on their knowledge and experiential wisdom[524].

Genetic Analysis of Human Variation

Classifying human populations is relevant in various epidemiological contexts. Several attempts have been made to represent the human population's genetic structure based on language, geographical divisions, racial or ethnic grouping[525]. Interpopulation genetic differences can be identified by gene polymorphism studies including SNP analyses[526]. Population based approaches are increasingly used to understand disease phenotypes. After completion of the human genome project understanding the role of genetic variations in determination of complex phenotypes that range from the shape of the nose to hypertension or CVD is a challenge. Correlating genotypes with phenotypes and differentiating populations on the basis of genetic or phenotypic characters may form the basis for evaluation of drug safety, efficacy and drug response, ultimately leading to designer medicine.

These phenotypes are not suitable for pedigree analysis, since susceptibility/resistance phenotypes of unexposed

---

[524] Patwardhan B. *et. al.,* Herbal remedies and bias against Ayurveda. Current Science, 2003: 84(9); 1165.

[525] Rosenberg NA, Pritchard JK, Weber JL, Cann HM, Kidd KK, Zhivotovsky LA, Feldman MW. Genetic structure of human populations. Science 2002; 298: 2381-85.

[526] Bamshad MJ, Wooding S, Watkins WS, Ostler CT, Batzer MA, Jorde LB. Population genetic structure and human classification. Am J Hum Genet 2003; 72: 578-89.

individuals are not accessible. For such diseases and other multifactorial phenotypes, population association analysis is employed to discover genetic effects. In such cases distortion of population genetic equilibrium (allele/genotype frequency, Hardy Weinberg Equilibrium and Linkage disequation LD) become tools of gene mapping. Association analysis involves either candidate genes or genome scans of DNA markers that track disease susceptibility by LD. One approach is screening of candidate genes for common SNPs in coding regions, in introns, in untranslaterd regions, upstream regulatory regions or promoter regions and even flanking microsatellites or short tandem repeats (STRS)[527].

The goal of this work is to define the nature of variation in human genes, as well as to provide a catalogue of gene polymorphisms for association studies. 106 genes whose protein products have roles in CVD, type II diabetes and schizophrenia were used for screening for variation in samples including Europeans, Africans, Americans, African Pygmies and Asians with average of 114 chromosomes screened for each gene where distribution of SNPs were seen in one of the subgroups[528].

Population association analysis involving candidate genes or random genome scans could also be used for drug efficacy and drug response analysis. The drugs are developed and safety tested with genetically homogenous animal systems. In clinical trials, they are tested in genetically heterogeneous human populations. Clinicians for similarly heterogeneous human patient populations

---

[527] Brahmachari S. K *et. al.*, CAG repeat instability at SCA2 locus: anchoring CAA interruptions and linked SNPs. Human Molecular Genetics 2001;10 (21) 2437-2446.

[528] Cargill *et. al.*, (1999) Characterization of single nucleotide polymorphism in coding regions of human genes. Nature Genetics 22, 231-237.

subsequently prescribe the drugs that make it to the market. Pharmacogenomics describes genomics based technologies to optimize the therapeutic efficacy of drugs through identification and characterization of genetic differences in target patient's populations[529] Recent papers have shown the feasibility of classifying humans into categorical populations from their genotypes with the claim that human races are biologically meaningless[530].

Microsatellites for Studying Genetic Variation

Microsatellites are tandem repeats of simple sequences that occur abundantly and at random throughout most eukaryotic genomes. They display considerable polymorphism due to variation in the number of repeat units. This polymorphism is sufficiently stable to be of use in genetic analyses. Microsatellites are therefore ideal markers for constructing high-resolution genetic maps in order to identify susceptibility loci involved in common genetic diseases. Neutral microsatellite markers have been used to infer genetic clusters for a heterogeneous population used in drug trial. The cytochromes P450 (CYP) catalyze the metabolism of numerous exogenous and endogenous molecules. Association of host risk factors such as germ line polymorphisms can contribute to genetic variations that cause differential drug metabolisms. Hence hosts carry an altered risk of treatment response. Consistent with this hypothesis, ethnic variation among the population throughout the world has shown significant alterations in genetic polymorphisms in P450. The frequencies of Drug

---

[529] Chicurel ME, Dalma-Weiszhausz DD. Microarrays in pharmacogenomics—advances and future promise. Pharmacogenomics 2002; 3 (5): 589-601

[530] Wilson JF, Weale ME, Smith AC, Gratrix F, Fletcher B, Thomas M, Bradman N, Goldstein DB. Population genetic structure of variable drug response. Nature Genetics 2001; 29: 265-69.

Metabolizing Enzyme loci (DME Loci) across the inferred clusters were assessed. It shows that commonly used ethnic labels such as black, Caucasian and Asian are insufficient and inaccurate descriptions of human genetic structure[531] Any such approach to human disease genetics will require an understanding of human gene variation. Sequence variation in human genes has been studied in limited way.

HLA Gene Polymorphism

Human major Histocompatibility complex (MHC) molecules are called human leukocyte antigens (HLA). It is well known that several HLA genes exhibit an extremely high degree of polymorphism and found to be polymorphic in various ethnic groups. In modern medicine, numerous chronic diseases are known to have an immunogenetic basis for cause and/or severity. It is well established that susceptibility and/or resistance to certain diseases is primarily associated with genes encoding peptide-presenting HLA molecules[532]. Type I diabetes, narcolepsy, coeliac disease (CD), ankylosing spondylitis (AS) and rheumatoid arthritis (RA) have each been clearly associated with specific class I or class II HLA genes. Association between HLA alleles and disease is usually quantified by typing HLA alleles expressed by individuals with the disease and healthy population. Relative risk can be calculated by comparing their frequencies of alleles. Analysis of population specific distribution of HLA alleles has proved to be important in finding out disease susceptibility or resistance in ethnic groups[533]. The extensive polymorphism

---

[531] Hearne *et. al.,* (1992) Microsatellites for linkage analysis of genetic traits TIG 8 (8) 288-294

[532] Nepom G T: Class II antigens and disease susceptibility. Annu Rev Med 1995;46:17- 25.

[533] Ritika Jaini, Gurvinder Kaur, Narinder K. Mehra: Heterogeneity of HLA-DRB1*04 and Its Associated Haplotypes in the North Indian Population. Human Immunology 2002;63:24-29.

of the HLA system also has useful applications in the study of the origin, evolution and migration patterns of human populations. Across various populations, HLA varies widely.

Diseases in Ayurveda are described in terms of imbalance in the 'tridoshas'. Individual constitution or '*Prakriti*' determines what kind of disorders one is prone to. Ayurveda considers that specific *Prakritis* are associated with specific disorders. We believe that Prakriti, disease proneness and HLA gene polymorphism will have some association. A broad based population analysis comparing these associations in different racial and ethnic groups should be especially informative to define more clearly these genetic interactions.

Ayu Genomics as a Tool for Classifying Human Population

Every individual is different. What determines the 'individuality' of a person? How do we identify genotypes associated with phenotypes and classify the human population? Systematic surveys of genetic variation form the basis for determination of population frequencies, genetic linkage studies and association studies relating genotype with phenotypes of interest to answer some of these questions. Genotypic or phenotypic classification of human populations is important in various epidemiological contexts: for better understanding disease[534], drug response[535,536] and others. Current classification of human

---

[534] Pearson ER, Starkey BJ, Powell RJ, Gribble FM, Clark PM and Hattersley AT. Genetic cause of hyperglycaemia and response to treatment in diabetes, The Lancet 2003; 362, (9392), 1275-1281.

[535] Meyer UA. Pharmacogenetics and adverse drug reactions, The Lancet 2000; 356 (9242), 667-1671.

[536] Kirchheiner J, Nickchen K, Bauer M, Wong ML, Licinio J, Roots I, Brockmoller. Pharmacogenetics of antidepressants and antipsychotics: the contribution of allelic variations to the phenotype of drug response. J Mol Psychiatry 2004; 9 (5), 442-473.

populations is broadly based on ethnicity, geographical location, language or self reported ancestry. However, such commonly used ethnic labels are inaccurate representations of genetic clusters and do not reflect underlying genetic make up[22]. The inability to explore such relationships is attributed to the complexity of human demographic history, which gives rise to neither an obvious natural clustering scheme, nor an obvious appropriate degree of resolution[537].

The Human Genome Project has revealed the complexity in the relationship between genotype and phenotype. Identifying specific phenotypic features and correlating them with genotypes constitute the basic program of phenomics[538]. A Proposed Human Phenome Project anticipates efforts to create comprehensive phenotypic data sets from different populations to find broad based genomic representation[539]. However there is no consensus on how to define phenotypes and which phenotypic features are to be included in the database. Classifying human populations thus remains a major challenge to biomedical sciences[540]. We explored *Ayurveda*, a traditional Indian System of Medicine for this purpose.

Prakriti is specific for each individual. It is said to be determined at the time of conception and remains unaltered during the lifetime i.e. in modern terms by the recombination of zygotic DNA from sperm and ovum. *Prakriti* specific treatment including prescription of

---

[537] Editorial, Nature Genetics 2001; 29, 239 – 240.

[538] Scriver CR. After the genome-the phenome? J Inherit Metab Dis. 2004; 27 (3): 305-17.

[539] Freimer N, Sabatti, C. The human phenome project. Nature Genetics 2003; 34: 15-21.

[540] Li-Ling. Human phenome based on traditional Chinese medicine- A solution to congenital syndromology. Am J Chinese Med 2003; 31 (6): 991-1000.

medications, diet and lifestyle is a distinctive feature of *Ayurveda*. We hypothesize that *Prakriti* has genetic connotation that could provide a tool for classifying human population based on broad phenotype clusters. We hypothesize that human phenome based on *Ayurveda* could provide an appropriate approach. Specifically, there could be a genetic basis for the three major constitutions (*Prakriti*) described in *Ayurveda*. The *Prakriti* classification is based on differences in physical, physiological and psychological characteristics and is independent of racial, ethnic or geographical considerations. It may provide an appropriate means of classifying phenotypes to be considered collectively for genotyping. As a pilot study to test the hypothesis, we evaluated 76 subjects both for their *Prakriti* and HLA DRB1 types. The genomic DNA was extracted using a standard protocol. Subsequently, HLA DRB1 typing was done by low-resolution Polymerase Chain Reaction- Sequence Specific Primers (PCR-SSP) and Oligonucleotide Probes (PCR- SSOP). We observed a reasonable correlation between HLA type and *Prakriti* types. Complete absence of HLA DRB1*02 allele in *Vata* and HLA DRB1* 13 in *Kapha* types remain significant observations with c2 = 4.715 and $p < 0.05$. HLA DRB1* 10 had higher allele frequency in *Kapha* type as compared to *Pitta* and *Vata* types. The homologous relation of tridosha to human genetic structure needs to be studied more for validation. If validated, our hypothesis would have far reaching implications for pharmacogenomics, modern genetics, human health and *Ayurveda*.

Reference

Patwardhan B. *et al.* JACM 2005

□□□

15 Ethnoinformatics and Ayu Soft

Very few traditional systems have a fair level of documentations in place. Most of the little traditions, the flow of knowledge is mainly through word of mouth, however, the great traditions such as Ayurveda and Traditional Chinese Medicine do have a good level of documentation. For instance, Ayurveda means science of life in Sanskrit and aims at holistic management of health and disease. It remains one of the most ancient medical systems widely practiced in Indian subcontinent and has a sound philosophical, experiential and experimental basis[541]. *Charak Samhita* and *Sushrut Samhita* (100-500 B.C.) are main Ayurvedic classics, which describe of over 700 botanicals along with their classification, pharmacological and therapeutic properties[542,543]. A classic diagnostic text *Madhav Nidana* includes over 5000 signs and symptoms. During the course of evolution and years actual practice, the interpretation of such documents developed different schools of thoughts and resulted in wide variations in

---

[541] Valiathan MS. The Legacy of Caraka, Orient Longman, 2003, Chennai India,.

[542] Charak Samhita, Translation 1995, Caukhambha Orientalia, Varanasi, India.

[543] Gogate V.M. Ayurvedic Pharmacology and Therapeutics of Medicinal Plants,2000, Bharatiya Vidya Bhavan's SPARC, Mumbai.

understandings. Similar situation also exists in other systems including TCM. These differences often raise issues related to authenticity and correctness of Traditional Knowledge (TK). Thus systematic documentation, interpretations and harmonization of concepts and practices remain a major challenge in most of the systems of TM. Many governments, professional and community organizations have undertaken such documentation and harmonization exercises. Projects like Traditional Medicine Knowledge Digital Library, AyuSoft, Triskandha Kosha and Medicinal Plants Database of FRLHT are attempting systematic documentation of Ayurveda in India[544]. Other databases such as The NAPRALERT (NAtural PRoducts ALERT) developed by Professor Norman Farnsworth contain bibliographic and factual data on natural products, including information on the pharmacology, biological activity, taxonomic distribution, ethno-medicine and chemistry of plant, microbial, and animal (including marine) extracts. Another project relates to the Global IP, Benefit Sharing and Traditional Medicine Database. It is being developed as a component of the Global Information Hub on Integrated Medicine from the work of the Commonwealth Working Group (CWG) on Traditional and Complementary Health Systems, now directed by the Malaysian Ministry of Health. This Information Hub is planning to create a network of legal centers, scholars and NGOs working together to develop a comprehensive legislative and policy review, information resource and exchange on issues pertaining to IP rights over traditional medical knowledge and the use of medicinal plants[545].

---

544 TKDL project of CSIR, AyuSoft project of CDAC/MICT Government of India.

545 Gerard Bodeker, Traditional (i.e. Indigenous) and Complementary Medicine in the Commonwealth: New Partnerships Planned With the Formal Health Sector, Journal of Alternative & Complementary Medicine 1999; 5, 97.

Other than such efforts, there is limited systematic documentation of TM knowledge and practices.

AyuSoft: A Decision Support System

Ayurveda is a holistic time tested Indian system of healing. India has a rich potential of traditional wisdom like Ayurveda. Globalization has led to increasing demand for Ayurveda. This needs integration of ancient wisdom and emerging technologies.The domain is vast and spread across various ancient texts. In-depth analysis of domain knowledge with integrated multidimensional view from all aspects is the needed. Understanding of Ayurveda is restricted due to language factor. Unbiased authentic understanding and its applications in clinical practice are required.

"AyuSoft is a vision of converting classical Ayurvedic texts into comprehensive, authentic, intelligent and interactive knowledge repositories with complex analytical tools". Its cutting-edge Features include: integrated system offering multiple interconnected applications under the same umbrella with systematic examination tool as per classical Ayurvedic guidelines. Investigations, Case Analysis etc. according to practical clinical needs and research challenges is possible.

It provides a High End Query Database with Multidimensional search utility to address heterogeneous needs of various user categories like Hospitals, Practitioners, Researchers including a Common Man and offers human expert analysis with human-independent analysis for treatment, medicine, plants, and substances. The current version of AyuSoft is based on the logic extracted from over 25,000 sutras from four major classical texts of Ayurveda. AyuSoft intends to be used as a decision support system for medical practitioners, students and researchers.

Applications as well as data can be plugged into AyuSoft to help you customize the tool to your specific needs. Aided by automated data loading and customized textual and graphical report generation capabilities, this unique tool will offer unparalleled functional flexibility and ease of navigation.

Thus, AyuSoft focuses on data mining wherein several databases interact with each other through the controlling computational engine enabling the users to act upon the useful information extracted from the enormous amount of available data.

Disease Diagnosis and Treatment based on signs-symptoms and causative factors provides probable diagnosis and specific treatment in form of formulations, single drugs, therapeutic procedures, and diet and lifestyle advice. Precise diagnosis up to specific conditions and subtypes of diseases is possible. Display of probable diseases based on probability and weightage along with detailed analytical study of pathogenesis is also possible. Specific treatment to specific conditions and subtypes of diseases are suggested. Multidimensional treatment includes formulations; herbs, procedures, diet and lifestyle considering indications and contraindications with common treatment for concomitant diseases are provided.

Prakriti Assessment Tool

Prakriti (constitution) is unique concept of Ayurveda that explains individuality and has role in prevention, diagnosis and treatment of diseases. It expresses unique trait of an individual that is defined by specific and permanent composition of *Dosha* (primary elements) at conception. Based on constitution assessed, diet and lifestyle advice is also suggested. Prakriti on Physical level is 'Dosha Prakriti' and psychological level is 'Maanas Prakriti'. Prakriti assessment is part of ten-point evaluation of an individual and helps physician to suggest diet and lifestyle to retain health. It is also important for diagnosis and selection of drugs for specific treatment. *Dhaatusaarataa* assessment defines status of *Dhaatu* (basic tissues). It is interpreted as excellent (Saara) and deprived (Asaara). Physician can speculate probable diseases and can suggest treatment accordingly.

Extensive questionnaire specific to age group and gender covers history, anatomical, physiological, psychological assessment with practical options to each question. Physician can modify weightage of each parameter. Diet & Lifestyle advice based on constitution, age specific questionnaire for old, adult, child & infant; analytical charts, graphs for better quantitative understanding; detail help for question and Prakriti, Saarataa data is made available for further research and correlations.

AyuSoft also provides Multimedia based Encyclopedia with Digitalized compendia and authentic glossary with search facility in English and Sanskrit. Elaborations of different aspects of Ayurveda with multimedia support; Articles on Ayurveda by stalwarts of Ayurveda; Video clips of therapeutic procedures; Images of herbs, instruments, diseases etc. are provided. A reporting tool for the user to search the data store based on his custom queries is very useful. Multidimensional complex search of signs, symptoms, causative factors, diseases, herbs, formulation, therapeutic procedures, diet, lifestyle, treatment principles and specific treatment options could be searched.

Patient Information Management System (PIMS) will help the user to capture and store complete case details of the patient. This helps to document and analyze clinical data. It assists extensive clinical examination and facilitates documentation of investigations, diagnosis, treatment etc. It covers all practical needs from patient registration, case taking, follow up and prescriptions; documentation of modern diagnosis, signs-symptoms, causative factors, diet, lifestyles, investigations, images and audio-video files etc. Wide-ranging clinical examination with contemporary parameters; customized lists of diagnosis, formulations, signs-symptoms, causative factors, diet, lifestyles and investigations; Automatic generation of certificates, prescription report etc. and Import and Export of patient's case for advice from other Physician can be obtained.

Case analysis is multidimensional analytical tool for research. Various clinical parameters along with investigations could be explored, correlated for statistical analysis. Extensive analysis of clinical data is useful for clinical trials, basic research, multiple correlations, which helps in evidence based research.

The system will be available in 3 variants: Shrink wrapped desktop application; Integrated solution for Intranet and Web-based integrated solution. AyuSoft Development team consists of IT professionals and Ayurveda experts of national as well as international repute. Collaborating agencies of AyuSoft are: Centre for Development of Advanced Computing, Pune, India; Interdisciplinary School of Health Sciences, and Department of Ayurveda, University of Pune; Jnanaprabodhini, Pune, India.

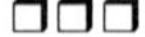

16 Systems Approaches and Reverse Pharmacology

The traditional medicines are actually used in human for number of years and therefore its clinical existence comes as a presumption. However, for bringing more objectivity and also to confirm traditional claims, systematic clinical trials are necessary. In Ayurvedic medicine research, clinical experiences, observations or available data becomes a starting point. In conventional drug research it comes at the last. Thus, the drug discovery based on Ayurveda follows a 'Reverse Pharmacology' path[546].

Nevertheless, all the critical Pharmacopoeial tests such as dissolution time, microbial, pesticide and heavy metals contamination etc. must be in accordance with global standards. It is important to ensure that all the Ayurvedic medicine manufacture is in accordance with Current Good Manufacturing Procedures for herbal products[547,548]. There

---

546 Vaidya A.D.B., Vaidya R.A., Nagaral S.I. Ayurvedaaa and a different level of evidence: From Lord Macaulay to Lord Walton (1835-2001 AD), Journal of Association of Physicians India (JAPI), 2001; 49:534-537 and Approach Paper, New Millennimum Indian Technology Leadership Initiative Herbal Drug Development Program, CSIR New Delhi, 2002.

547 Good manufacturing practices: Supplementary guidelines for manufacture of Herbal Medicinal products In: WHO expert committee on specifications for pharmaceutical preparations. Thirty fourth report. Geneva, World Health Organization, 1996,Annex8 (WHO technical Series, no 863). P.134-139.

548 Verpoorte R and Mukherjee P. GMP for Botanicals, businesshorizons.com, 2003.

have been concerns about quality standards and safety issues of herbal medicines[549]. The need for new regulations for botanical medicines has also been frequently stressed and some such regulations are coming in force in different parts of the world[550,551].

Systems Approach

Traditional medicines have been developed through real life experiences and direct observations in people with diseases and representhighly complex biological systems. Typical drug discovery pipeline include preclinical studies on animal models, cells and tissue screens High throughput assays capable of interrogating individual molecular targets with a number of compounds speed up screening process enormously. Yet, numbers of new chemical/molecular entities that are approved are declining[552]. This situation calls for critical assessment of current strategies where only new chemical entities are valued as potential new drugs. Molecular biological technology is primarily used for defining molecular targets and for creating new miniaturized screening tests. Such reductionism where whole organism is broken down to groups of cells, subcells, molecules, molecular interactions undermines importance of the whole system. While interacting with each other macromolecules form complex networks organized into systems with properties that extend beyond individual

---

[549] Straus S. Herbal Medicines – What's in the Bottle? NEJM 2002: 347(25);1997-1998.

[550] Legal Status of Traditional Medicine- A Worldwide Review, W.H.O. Geneva 2001.

[551] Marcus D and Grollman A. Botanical Medicines – The need for new regulations, NEJM 2002: 347(25); 2073-2076.

[552] Butcher E.C., Berg E.L., Kunkel E.J., 2004. Systems biology in drug discovery. Nature Biotechnology, 22(10) 1253-1259.

functions. Systems biology attempts to provide predictive models of behavior of such molecular systems to identify such functional interactions[553]. Ludwig Von Bertalanffy who proposed systems theory states 'Compared to the analytical procedure of classical science with resolution into component elements and one-way or linear causality as basic category, the investigation of organized wholes of many variables requires new categories of interaction, transaction, organization, teleology'[554].

Current strategy of drug development of single target, single compound, is based on a super reductionism that involves mostly tests of compounds at the molecular level assays. This approach is not suitable for studies on traditional medicines. A more holistic approach using systems biology seems much more suited to proof efficacy and to obtain information that might lead to understanding the mode of action.

Systems approach or science of wholeness is the unique philosophy of Ayurveda. When multiple cell types and diverse pathways contribute to the disease, a single molecule may not be effective in modulation of multiple targets and such conditions require combination therapy. Modern medicine has also developed combination of drugs for addressing more than one therapeutic target[555]. Herbal extracts represent combinatorial chemistry of nature with

---

[553] Gannon F. 2005. Welcome to molecular systems biology. EMBO Report. 6(4), 291.

Gillis N.C. 2001. Biomedical Science and Herbal Medicine: A Reluctant but Necessary Alliance. FASEB Newsletter 34, (1).

[554] Ludwig von Bertalanffy (1968). General System Theory: Foundations, Development, Applications New York: George Braziller.

[555] Morphy RK Corinne and Rankovic 2004. From magic bullets to designed multiple ligands. Drug Discovery Today 9 (15) 641-51.

vast array of chemical compounds that can deal with multiple targets simultaneously leading to synergistic systems effect. Considerable experimental evidence is now built up to support use of molecular technology such as microarrays for testing herbal drugs that work in system to arrive at their targets.

The genomics, proteomics and now metabonomics take the center stage in science. Earlier the drugs were created in within the confines of a chemical paradigm of medicine and drug therapy. We are now witnessing the entry of a new informational paradigm into medicine that is most prominently represented by proteomics, metabonomics sciences. Metabonomics is a systems approach for studying in vivo metabolic profiles, which promises to provide information on drug toxicity, disease processes and gene function at several stages in the DD process. It uses spectroscopic methods like nuclear magnetic resonance (NMR), liquid chromatography mass spectroscopy (LCMS) and gas chromatography mass spectroscopy (GCMS) methods for identifying and characterizing certain metabolic changes in human, then integrating the data out come by bioinformatics software and creating a metabolic profile for a single individual. Such integration of data types will also pave the way to understanding the relationships between gene function and metabolic control in health and disease. Systems Biology (SB) thus offers the computational integration of data generated by the suite of genetic, transcriptomic, proteomic and metabonomic platforms to understand function through different levels of biomolecular organization. This offers exciting new prospects for determining the causes of human disease and finding possible cures. Certainly the judicious use of 'omics' data should give new insights and opportunities for the DD process and for understanding drug toxicology.

This paradigm will bring two important changes in the therapy of diseases. First, science will mature to such a degree that it will study complex genomes and their functionality in complex organisms such as humans. Therefore, results from these studies no longer have to be translated into the context of medicine: they are already within this context. Secondly, drug therapy that used to be largely symptomatic, will now aim at targets emerging from the system that are closer to the causes of diseases. Therapeutic progress, which used to be indirect, conjectural and coincidental, is about to become more directed, definitive and intentional. The future drug discovery will be more often based on intent rather than coincidence. Proper bioprospecting of medicinal sources will still remain an important factor.

However, despite the call from the Food and Drug Administration (FDA) for an increase in science-based drug development and the recognition within the industry of the productivity challenges, there is only sporadic activity directly in line with the systems thinking presented here. Proof-of-principle studies are currently being undertaken, but no critical path success has yet emerged. From a cost-benefit point of view, the full incorporation of systems thinking into the pharmaceutical value chain will substantially increase the cost in short term. The implementation of such a new concept over the entire process can only take place gradually, given the existing infrastructures that might need to be changed, the current development pipelines and the regulatory constraints. The analytical platforms necessary to undertake systems approaches are not inexpensive, nor trivial, to implement. Furthermore, the effort to establish quality-controlled methods to acquire, store, integrate and interpret datasets from different analytical platforms is substantial and the task of obtaining high-quality biological samples from animal and clinical studies is time- and human-resource consuming. The current need of the industry is a cost-effective, fast track approach for DD[6].

Reverse Pharmacology (RP)

A new chemical entity (NCE) travels a path from laboratories to clinics, which involve target identification, lead identification, lead optimization, preclinical studies, and then four phases of the clinical trials. Time involved in this NCE approach is about 6-8 years with an investment of about 800 million in 2004 to 1.2 billion in 2006 and still rising. The DD process is becoming more and more complex and capital-intensive and such companies remain 'target rich' but 'lead poor', with lead discovery as a greater bottleneck. In such a situation, industrialization of DD process is underway. Although high throughput screening (HTS) and combinatorial chemical synthesis are explored with great hope, general experience tells us that in most companies the investments in these technologies have not reaped rewards in new lead discovery as expected. Despite technological advances, genomics and bioinformatics predictions, actually the number of new molecular (chemical and biological) entities has dropped during the year 2002 to less than 20/year. FDA reported 75 % of the NCE failing in phase III which causing huge losses. Recently ragaglitazar of Novo failed in Phase III. Approaches like RP helps in reducing three major bottlenecks of costs, time and toxicity

Reverse Pharmacology, as an academic discipline, can be perceived to comprise of three phases, as described under:

Experiential robust documentation of clinical observations of the biodynamic effects of standardized Ayurvedic drugs by meticulous record keeping. Exploratory studies for tolerability, drug-interactions, dose-range finding in ambulant patients of defined subsets of the disease and paraclinical studies in relevant *in vitro* and *in vivo* models to evaluate the target-activity. Experimental studies, basic and clinical, at several levels of biological organization, to identify and validate the reverse pharmacological correlates of Ayurvedic drug safety and efficacy. Such a creative research endeavor requires an excellent teamwork by multisystem and multidisciplinary experts. Reverse pharmacology, for drug development, has been highly productive and cost-effective too in the recent past. Globally, this approach has now generated greater interest in Ayurveda and Pharmacology. The scope of reverse pharmacology is to understand the mechanisms of action, at multiple levels of biology and to optimize safety, efficacy and acceptability of the leads in NP, based on relevant science. In this approach as the candidate travels a reverse path from 'clinics to lab' rather than classical 'lab to clinics path'.

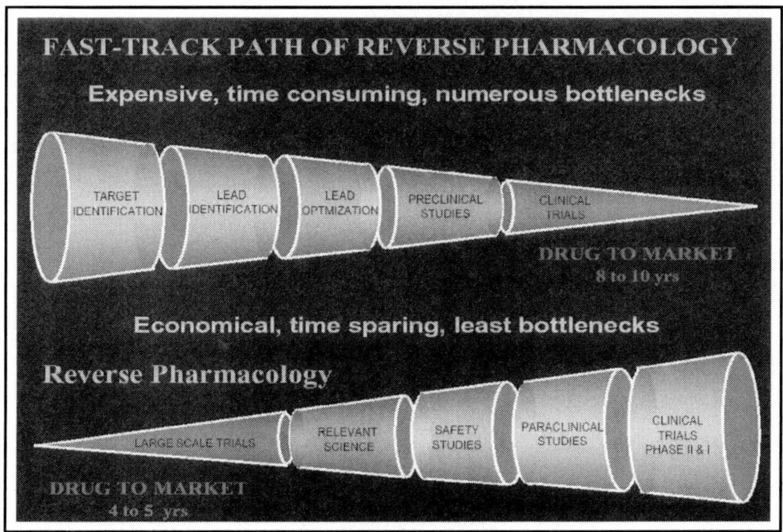

Reverse Pharmacology Path

Acual human use is the ultimate 'model' and in-depth investigation of the effects of drugs and the nature of disease progression is becoming ever more feasible because of advances in clinical biomarkers and SB. SB approach articulates - both structure of the system and components plays indispensable role forming symbiotic state of the system as a whole. Combining the RP and SB approach the DD for NP can be accelerated. We need to adopt such innovative approaches, models and designs in studying human subjects for establishing proof of mechanism and concept of natural drugs. We list some of the case studies emerging from this approach.

Case Studies

Rauwolfia serpentina (Sarpagandha)

Ganath Sen and Bose not only showed the antihypertensive effects of Sarpagandha but they were also astute clinicians to note certain side effects like parkinsonism, depression, gynecomastia, acid-peptic symptoms etc. It was only recently that, a Nobel Prize in Medicine and Physiology was given to those who validated and explained the actions by mechanistic correlates[7]. As a spin-off of the side effects of *Rauwolfia serpentina*, several new drugs were developed viz. L-dopa, antidepressants, bromoergocriptine, and H2-receptor blockers etc[8, 9, 10]. The alkaloids of *Rauwolfia serpentina*, reserpine and ajmalcine, have served as research tools in many experiments[11,12]. There are still some unanswered questions: does reserpine have more incidences of depression and/or extrapyramidal side effects than the standardized extract of the plant? It is worthwhile to apply combinatorial chemical methods for reserpine-derivatives, which do not cross the blood-brain barriers, so that depression is avoided as a side effect. The uptake of norepinephrine by isolated chromaffin granules, by inhibition of ATP-Mg^2 – dependent mechanism has to be studied freshly at the transcriptional level. The *kaphavatashamak* (anti-inflammatory) properties of the plant described in Ayurveda too need an investigation. Though reserpine is withdrawn globally, the extracts of the plant are used as Ayurvedic drugs. There is a need to conduct pharmacovigilance on Sarpagandha ghanavati.

Picrorrhiza kurroa (Kutki)

Late Vaidya Zandu Bhattji for the treatment of jaundice has popularized Arogyawardhani. A double-blind trial with Arogyawardhani Kutki and placebo was conducted in viral hepatitis[13,14]. As significant hepatoprotective effects were observed of Kutki, as in Arogyawardhani or as a single plant. Later, picrosides, the active principles of Kutki were also tested *in vivo* and *in vitro*[15-22]. Significant antioxidants as well as hydrocholeritic effects were noted for Kutiki[23]. These effects of hepatoprotection in CCl_4 and galactosamine[16] models are considered the pharmacological correlates of clinical actions. However, there is a need to study at the cellular and molecular levels how the water outflow in the biliary microcanaliculae is enhanced. CDRI has now developed a cucurbitacin-free extract of *P. kurroa* (Picroliv), which is now in Phase III trials. The plant also inhibits passive cutaneous anaphylaxis, as shown by Mahajani[24].

Commiphora wightii (Guggulu)

Guggulu is a major Ayurvedic drug and used widely and in diverse formulations. A monograph of all the major citations has been published. Hypolipidemic effects of guggulu were primarily discovered through reverse pharmacology mode. Antarkar, Satyavati, and Nityanand have done exetensive study on the hypolipidemic effect of guggulu[25, 26]. The product has been already marketed and widely used. However, the anti-arthritic effects of guggulu in clinic have been relatively less investigated. We have sizeable experiential and reverse pharmacological studies with standardized guggulu preparations[27]. Phase I study, long-term and large dose ambulant studies and have been conducted. The on-going studies at cellular and molecular levels have helped in evolving pharmacological correlates of clinically shown actions. The side-effects of guggulu have also been documented. The mechanisms of toxicity are yet to be studied. Guggulu can offer a platform for technological innovations in pharmaceutics, pharmacodynamics and pharmacokinetics. The use of guggulu as a homadravya [Sacrificial incense] in Shantikarma (sacrificial use) is currently being evaluated for the antimicrobial effects of the volatiles. Topical formulations of guggulu demand unique dermato-pharmacological reverse correlates. The statement found in the literature on different properties of fresh and old guggulu need additional clinical investigations–experiential and exploratory.

Use of Ayurvedic therapeutics in context of the modern medicine will give us many more insights into the newer targets in the disease pathogenesis and effects of the drugs. Blending the ancient wisdom and the modern science open up exiting fields where both can be benefited mutually adopting each others techniques.

Ethnopharmacology Approaches

Traditional medical doctors often apply a holistic approach in prescribing medicines to the patient. Each individual patient gets his own optimalized medicine, usually a mixture of different ingredients. To develop the natural product DD means to establish a proof of efficacy through defined experiments to benefit the mankind. That proof may not be as expected by the modern medicine doctors[28]. Traditional medicines can have a different kind of evidence where n = 1 study must be made mandatory. By n = 1 studies means a single patient should be studied for his response to the drug. The response can be measured either by pharmacodynamic or the traditional methods, developed and practiced by these traditional systems of medicine over ages. We need not focus our efforts directed only to the *in vitro* receptor binding assays to create evidence. We may loose out in doing so as plant may have thousands of chemical entities acting on in synergism to modify a disease. Thus we may not be able to locate the single chemical entity by out reductionist approach. For e.g. St. John's wort no single active compound has been found that can explain the proven clinical activity. Only *in vivo* screening designs will help us for herbal drug development.

Based on the traditional experiences drug development for herbal drugs can follow the different paths explained in the following chart-

First is the ethno medicine path based on observing the field use of the plants and then standardizing it for the activity e.g. tubocurarine isolated from *Curare* – commonly known as South American arrow poison. Another most adapted path is screening of the extracts in selected models, isolation of the active principles and then a modern drug, which enter a preclinical, clinical phase e.g. isolation of reserpine from *Rauwolfia serpentina*. Third path is the herbal product path of screening of extract in models and then testing the extract for its efficacy and safety in a clinical set up e.g. *Ganoderma lucidum* and *Hypericum perforatum*. The fourth path is the holistic path using the formulation mentioned in classical texts of Ayurveda and then evaluating its efficacy through pharmacoepidemological studies e.g. chavanprash. All the above paths are paths explored for years together with and have yielded blockbuster medicines. In spite of all these established approaches the contribution to drugs remained limited as the pharmaceutical companies refrained themselves from taking this field seriously. In addition, although botanical medications continued to be produced in every country, the clinical efficacy of these was usually not evaluated and the composition of these complex mixtures was only crudely analyzed. Thus the investments in DD for NP remained scares. This has resulted in the slow tracking of the NP DD. Then main reasons, which can be pointed out for the slow tracking are -

Failure to distinguish folklore from traditionally established systems like Ayurveda and TCM, lack of proper identity and Good Botanical Practices, improper experiential documentation, absence of Phase II dose searching, cultural prejudice for alien "science", emphasis on the reductionist path, and lack of political & financial support.

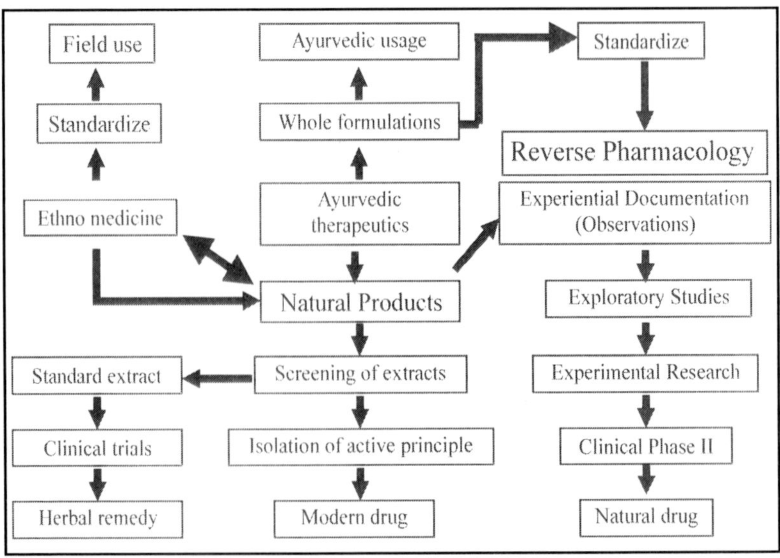

R & D Paths for Natural Products

Plants are tight compositional complex mixtures of chemicals and studying these mixtures itself is a challenge. We will require an open-ended approach, which will guide us from the traditional wisdom of Ayurveda to the current state-of-art developments in biology. Such an integrative and interdisciplinary approach can be the key to understand the breadth of the drug action and should be a crucial exercise to rescue the NP DD.

Ayurveda as a New Discovery Engine

Combining the strengths of the knowledge base of traditional systems such as Ayurveda with the dramatic power of combinatorial sciences and HTS will help in the generation of structure–activity libraries. Ayurvedic knowledge and experiential database can provide new functional leads to reduce time, money and toxicity - the three main hurdles in drug development. These records are particularly valuable, since effectively these medicines have been tested for thousands of years on people. Efforts are underway to establish pharmacoepidemiological evidence base regarding safety and practice of Ayurvedic medicines. Development of standardized herbal formulations is underway as an initiative of the Council for Scientific and Industrial Research (CSIR) New Millennium Indian Technology Leadership Initiative (NMITLI). Randomized controlled clinical trials for diabetes, rheumatoid and osteoarthritis, hepatoprotectives, and many other disorders have reasonably established clinical efficacy. A review of some exemplary evidence-based researches and approaches has now resulted in wider acceptance of Ayurvedic medicines. Thus the Ayurvedic knowledge database allows drug researchers to start from a well-tested and safe botanical material. With Ayurveda, the normal drug discovery course of 'laboratories to clinics' actually becomes from 'clinics to laboratories' - a true reverse pharmacology approach. Globally, there is a positive trend towards holistic health, integrative sciences, systems biology approaches in drug discovery and therapeutics that has remained one of the unique features of Ayurveda. A golden triangle consisting of Ayurveda, modern medicine and science will converge to form a real discovery engine that can result in newer, safer, cheaper and effective therapies. It will be in the interest of pharmaceutical companies, researchers and ultimately the global community to respect the traditions and build on their knowledge and experiential wisdom.

NMITLI – a Successful Experiment and Challenges Ahead

It was a need to time to initiate a National interdisciplinary networking effort for research on NP DD approaches. CSIR has taken a timely initiative and this project was named as NMITLI. The novelty of the proposal is in the integrative approach that encompasses reverse pharmacology, ethno medicine, herbal technology and systems-biology approach. The concept to product path will be essentially carried out through RP, but the standard elements of a global herbal product-dossier are addressed. This will help in generating wealth thorough intellectual property rights (IPR). The main deliverables of the project are to frame and undertake an approach for NP DD in India.

❑❑❑

17 Future Perspectives

Looking forward, it is clear that traditional and western medicine have the potential for rich collaboration that benefits both disciplines. There is growing interest in this partnership, as shown by the number of international journals now dedicated to such research, such as Journal of Ethnopharmacology, Complementary Therapies in Medicine, eCAM, Alternative Therapies in Health and Medicine, and the Journal of Alternative and Complementary Medicine. Even the WHO has taken note of the rich possibilities of the future of TM, having put out such documents as 'WHO General Guidelines for Methodologies on Research and Evaluation of Traditional Medicine' and 'WHO Guidelines on Good Agricultural and Collection Practices (GACP) for Medicinal Plants'. Despite this enthusiasm, there are several areas where the international community will need to focus their attention if the goal of integrating botanical medicines for the good of human health is to be reached.

Acquisition of Knowledge

Individuals, tribes, and healers currently hold a wealth of traditional medical knowledge. It is a formidable but necessary task to begin to collect and sort this information and verify the proposed health benefits. In this process, it is important that a basis of trust is build between those who wish to use TM and those who hold the information. Local healers must be empowered at every step of the acquisition process if this trust is to be developed.

To be of greatest benefit and to preserve indigenous knowledge, the information derived from botanical medicines should be cataloged in a standardized and accessible manner. The Convention on Biological Diversity urged nations to catalog information on botanical medicines both to preserve the knowledge and to allow local groups to benefit from their intellectual property[556]. For example, if germplasm banks are developed and maintained, it will ensure that future generations have access to currently available botanical specimens[557]. This example is highlights just one way to make traditional medical knowledge more accessible to a wide variety of interested people. The more effects that can be made to push for standardization and accessibility of traditional medical knowledge, the more that the global community stands to benefit.

Within this framework, it is important to keep in mind the intellectual property rights of the individuals who hold TM knowledge. Local groups and their collaborators should share both short and long term benefits of their partnership, even as far into the future as the discovery and commercialization of the drugs that result from TM. For the future, there is tremendous potential for the local stakeholders to push for research and treatments that result from TM to be relevant to the developing world.

---

[556] Soejarto, D.D. 2005 Ethnobotany/ethnopharmacology and mass bioprospecting: Issues on intellectual property and benefit-sharing. Journal of Ethnopharmacology 100 15–22

[557] Cordell, G.A. 1995. Changing strategies in natural products chemistry. Phytochemistry 40, 1585–1612.

Safety and Regulation

If botanical medicines are to gain prominence, their toxicity and safety profiles will have to be of highest priority. Even medicines that have been used traditionally will need evaluation on their interactions with other commonly used allopathic medicines. Beginning this research will require that standards for evaluating the safety and toxicity of herbal medicines are developed. A few of the many issues that will need to be addressed are potential contamination with heavy metals, insecticides, radioactivity and the like, batch-to-batch standardization, shelf life of the final product[558].

Safety evaluations can be even more complex for botanical medicines than for single target allopathic drugs, particularly because they don't fall into a well-established framework. The costs of this research are substantial; while the US National Institute of Health spends about 33% of their budget on testing the safety and efficacy of drugs within an allopathic framework, the US National Center for Complementary and Alternative Medicine spends as much as 80% of their budget to evaluate the same factors in traditional medicines. If a push can be made to implement universal standards for herbal medicines, perhaps these costs can be driven down.

WHO began the push for such standards, which focused on the importance of harmonizing terms used for botanical medicines, summarizing the issues for the development of research methodologies, improving the quality and value of research on TM, and providing appropriate evaluation methodologies to facilitate regulation and registration[559]. In the future, these guidelines

---

[558] Cordell, G.A. 2005 Some thoughts on the future of ethnopharmacology. Journal of Ethnopharmacology 100. 5–14

[559] WHO Traditional Medicine Strategy 2002-2005, WHO Geneva.

need to be turned into concrete standards with input from the myriad stakeholders. The proper use of traditional medical knowledge draws in individuals from many arenas: academic, corporate, state, and private, which will make intra-sectorial collaboration necessary.

Research

Worldwide, it has become clear that quality research is the main key to unlocking the benefits of traditional medicine. Once research guidelines are in place, there must be trained professionals to carry out the work and local research centers to serve as hubs for data collection. This will involve building the capacity of the local infrastructure and personnel. The principles of evidence-based research should be integrated into the research plans for traditional medicine. Training investigators, educating medical students, and building international research networks will all help to build up the capacity to perform research validating traditional medicine.

As research progresses, making it available is essential to avoid needless duplication of research. Organizations like the International Society of Complementary Medicine and Research, which is backed by the US, UK and Canada, seek to develop an international complementary and alternative medicine community to facilitate information flow[560]. Much as local groups must be integrated into the process of acquisition of traditional medical knowledge, they should be equal players in international research consortiums.

Technological advances will undoubtedly play a role in how traditional medical research is carried out in

[560] Lewith, George. 2006 Developing CAM Research Capacity for Complementary Medicine. eCAM 2006; 3(2)283–289

the future. Bioassays that involve automation and nanotechnology are increasingly common in medical research. Real-time PCR will allow for rapid identification of botanical materials. Microarray tools can help screen potential drugs for their impact on the genome. Proteomics tools will also permit rapid screening of botanical materials[561]. All future technologies must conform to standards of affordability and easy transport for field research.

Sustainability

One of the dangers of pursuing traditional medical knowledge on a global scale is the potential impact on local biodiversity. As mentioned by the WHO Fact sheet n. 134 on Traditional Medicine, "Growing herbal market and its great commercial benefit might pose a threat to biodiversity through over-harvesting of the raw material for herbal medicines and other natural health care products. These practices, if not controlled, may lead to the extinction of endangered species and the destruction of natural habitats and resources[562].

Special efforts need to be made to prevent the extinction of herbal medicines and the exhaustion of the local environment. Sustainable agricultural techniques should be introduced for cultivation and collection of botanical medicines to ensure future access to medicinal plants. In cases where illegal trade is playing a role in local environmental degradation, it will be necessary to increase surveillance and monitoring to ensure that an unlawful market for treatments does not skirt environmental regulations.

---

[561] Cordell, G.A. 2005 Some thoughts on the future of ethnopharmacology. Journal of Ethnopharmacology 100. 5–14

[562] WHO Fact sheet n. 134 on Traditional Medicine. May 2003.

Health Care Systems

From a public policy perspective, there is quite a bit that can be done to facilitate the use of traditional medicine. First and foremost, all of the research and policy work that is done in the name of traditional medicine must have the health of the people as its first priority. One of the most promising features of traditional medicine is that, if pursued correctly, it offers the possibility for individual nations to develop affordable treatments for their people. In addition, traditional healers have the potential to be effectors of great change in their communities. As the old adage says, a message to be effective at changing behavior, it has to be the right message delivered by the right messenger. In communities where the traditional healer is the healthcare provider, he can serve as a culturally accepted bridge between allopathy and traditional medicine[563]. In the end, it is the health of the people that stands to benefit.

Each nation will need to evaluate its healthcare needs to find the best combination of allopathic and traditional medicine. Nations need to start asking questions about integrating traditional medicine into their national health policy. What is the best balance of allopathy and traditional medicine to suit the health needs of the people? What combination of services will address the burden of diseases that affects the largest sector of people? Which treatments will be the most cost effective? Which are the most culturally acceptable? What needs to be done to assure that marginalized populations have their healthcare needs met? In addition to national policies, international funding organizations should ask similar questions about how to best involve traditional medicine in their health agendas.

---

[563] Ghodossou, Erick. AIDS in Africa: Scenarios for the Future. The Role of Traditional Medicine in Africa's Fight Against HIV/AIDS.

Currently, only 25 of the 191 member states of the WHO have a national traditional medicine/complementary and alternative medicine policy[564].

National healthcare policy will have to develop a framework to build their policy. Cooperation between allopathic and traditional medical systems will need to start with individual care providers and extend as far up as the policy-making bodies. Regulation can't occur unless traditional medicine and its care providers are officially recognized and registered. This recognition will allow traditional medicine care providers to integrate into the standard healthcare system more effectively. WHO Traditional Medicine Strategy also details the things that must be avoided when crafting a national healthcare policy that includes traditional medicine:

"Careful assessment has first to be made of the use and practice of TM/CAM in the relevant country and the most appropriate means of using TM/CAM therapies. National policies should benefit patients using TM/CAM therapies. They fail to provide this benefit if they are: unable to ensure the safety, efficacy, and quality of TM/CAM products and practices; unduly restrict the practice of TM/CAM; lead to higher health care costs; unjustifiably hinder patient treatment options; or reduce the ability of allopathic medicine practitioners to cross-refer patients" (WHO Traditional Medicine Strategy 2002-2005)

Globally, the coverage of health insurance is far from equitable, although it plays a role in access to different forms of healthcare. Those people who do have insurance are more likely to use services that are covered by their plans,

---

[564] Bodecker, Gerard. Oct 2002. A Public Health Agenda for Traditional, Complementary, and Alternative Medicine American Journal of Public Health I October 2002, Vol 92, No. 10.

which currently excludes traditional medicine in many cases. In the context of developing countries, insurance typically covers allopathic treatments that have been proven safe and effective. The majority of people who fall outside this scope are left with poor and unregulated medical services. Health insurance programs will need to address the integration of traditional medicine into their schemes with a focus on making safe services available to poorer segments of society.

The future possibilities for the integration of traditional medicine place us at an exciting juncture. The world truly stands to benefit from the wealth of knowledge that is a part of traditional medicine. On the other hand, traditional medicine offers the impetus to move forward to western medicine, to try and understand the complexity of a different system of healing. Building an understanding of how and why traditional medicines work can only help to elucidate the equally complex factors that affect health. For those people involved, it may become the case that they have to turn their attention towards advocacy and ethics, looking at their work as a catalyst for international development and collaboration. In developing a vision for the future, the integration of traditional provides the international community with a unique opportunity to look at health as a right that can and must be provided to all segments of humanity. With this exciting possibility as the premise, it is time to truly begin to work on bringing traditional medicine and allopathic medicine together into a partnership to create an equitable system of health.

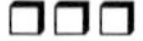

Glossary and Abbreviations

AAAS : American Association for the Advancement of Science (AAAS). In addition to publishing *Science* and other science-related publications, hosting scientific conferences and meetings, and helping scientists advance their careers, AAAS undertakes numerous programs and activities that promote science to the public and monitor issues which affect the scientific community.

ADR : Adverse Drug Reactions. Medicines can treat or prevent illness and disease. However, sometimes medicines can cause problems. These problems are called adverse drug reactions.

AIDS : Acquired Immuno-Deficiency Syndrome is caused by infection with the human immunodeficiency virus HIV-1. The HIV virus infects cells in the body that fight infection.

AYUSH : Department of Ayurveda, Yoga and Naturopathy, Unani, Siddha and

Homeopathy. Formerly known as Department of Indian System of Medicine and Homeopathy (ISM&H). Ministry of Health and Family Welfare, Govt. of India, established AYUSH to promote ISM & H.

CAM : Complementary and Alternative medicine is a group of diverse medical and health care systems, practices, and products that are not presently considered to be part of conventional medicine.

CBD : Convention on Biological Diversity. The three goals of the CBD are to promote the conservation of biodiversity, the sustainable use of its components, and the fair and equitable sharing of benefits arising out of the utilization of genetic resources. This Convention on Biological Diversity was negotiated under the auspices of the United Nations Environment Program (UNEP).

CCRAS : Central Council for Research in Ayurveda and Siddha (CCRAS) is an apex body for the formulation, coordination and development of research in Ayurveda & Siddha on scientific lines. It was established in March 1978 after reorganization of CCRIM&H. The Minister of Health & Family Welfare, Govt. of India, is the President of the Governing Body of the Council.

CIPIH : Commission on Intellectual Property, Innovation and Public Health was established by the World Health Assembly in 2003 to collect data and proposals from the different factors involved and produce an analysis of intellectual property rights, innovation, and public health, including the question of appropriate funding and incentive mechanisms for the creation of new medicines and other products against diseases that disproportionately affect developing countries.

CMC : Chemistry, Manufacturing and Controls.

CSM : Committee on the Safety of Medicines (CSM) is one of the independent advisory committees established under the Medicines Act which advises the UK Licensing Authority on the quality, efficacy and safety of medicines in order to ensure that appropriate public health standards are met and maintained.

CSIR : Council for Scientific and Industrial Research (CSIR), India, is an autonomous body registered under the Societies Registration Act, 1860 with a wide-ranging charter for promotion and development of science and technology. Established in 1942, by Govt. of India, CSIR has a network of 40 laboratories and 80 Field Extension Centers spread all over India.

CGMP : Current Good Manufacturing Procedures are set of current scientifically sound methods, practices or principles that are implemented & documented during product development and production to ensure consistent manufacture of safe, pure and potent products.

CWG : Commonwealth Working Group is an association of 53 countries. It's 1.8 billion citizens; about 30 percent of the world's population are drawn from the broadest range of faiths, races, cultures and traditions. Members range from vast countries like Canada to small island states like Malta.

DBT : Department of Biotechnology is established by Govt. of India as a separate Department under the Ministry of Science and Technology in 1986 for providing new impetus to the development of the field of modern biology and biotechnology in India.

DSHEA : The Dietary Supplement Health and Education Act of 1994 was enacted by Congress following public debate concerning the importance of dietary supplements in promoting health, the need for consumers to have access to current and accurate information about supplements, and controversy over the Food and Drug Administration's regulatory approach to this product category.

DST : Department of Science and Technology was established in May 1971 by Govt. of India with the objective of promoting new areas of Science & Technology and to play the role of a nodal department for organizing, coordinating and promoting S&T activities in the country.

EBM : Evidence-Based Medicine/Healthcare is looked upon as a new paradigm, replacing the traditional medical paradigm, which is based on authority. It is dependent on the use of randomized controlled trials, as well as systematic reviews (of a series of trials) and meta-analysis, although it is not restricted to these. There is also an emphasis on the dissemination of information, as well as its collection, so that the evidence can reach clinical practice.

EMEA : European Medicines Evaluation Agency is a decentralized body of the European Union with headquarters in London. EMEA is an agency to contribute to the protection and promotion of public and animal health by mobilizing scientific resources from throughout the European Union to provide high quality evaluation of medicinal products, to advise on research and development programs and to provide useful and clear information to users and health professionals.

EU : European Union is a union of twenty-five independent states based on the European Communities and founded to enhance political, economic and social co-operation. Formerly known as European Community (EC) or European Economic Community (EEC).

FDA : Food and Drug Administration of US is a federal science-based law enforcement agency mandated to protect public health and safety. FDA is responsible for protecting the public health by assuring the safety, efficacy, and security of human and veterinary drugs, biological products, medical devices, our nation's food supply, cosmetics, and products that emit radiation.

GCP : Good Clinical Practices is a standard for design, conduct, performance, monitoring, audit, recording, analyses and reporting of clinical trials that the data and reported results are credible and accurate, and that the rights, and confidentiality of trial subjects are protected.

GLP : Good Laboratory Practices.

GMP : Good Manufacturing Practices.

GRA : Global Research Alliance represents the combined knowledge and experience of nine of the world's leading knowledge-intensive technology organizations. The alliance will explore ways of exploiting the resources of the participatory members to the benefits of the society at large.

FRLHT : Foundation for Revitalization of Local Health Traditions is a non-government organization situated at Bangalore, India, and working towards conservation of India's traditional medicinal heritage.

HIV : Human Immunodeficiency Virus (refer to AIDS).

HPLC : High Performance Liquid Chromatography is a popular method of analysis. Modern HPLC has many applications including separation, identification, purification, and quantification of various compounds.

HPTLC : High Performance Thin Layer Chromatography is a sophisticated and automated form of TLC. The main difference between HPTLC and TLC is particle and pore size of sorbents.

ICH : The International Conference on Harmonization of Technical Requirements for Registration of Pharmaceuticals for Human Use; is a unique project that brings together the regulatory authorities of Europe, Japan and the United States and experts from the pharmaceutical industry in the three regions to discuss scientific and technical aspects of product registration.

ICMR : The Indian Council of Medical Research is a apex body in India for the formulation, coordination and promotion of biomedical research, is one of the oldest medical research bodies in the world.

IK : Indigenous Knowledge can refer to the knowledge belonging to a specific ethnic group, for example: 'Indigenous knowledge is the local knowledge that is unique to a given culture or society. It is the basis for local-level decision-making in agriculture, health care, food preparation, education, natural resource management, and a host of other activities in rural communities.'

IP : Intellectual Property is a property that enjoys legal protection and stems from the exercise of the mind. Includes patents, trademarks, copyright, design protection and some minor rights.

IPR : Intellectual Property Rights are Creative ideas and expressions of the human mind that possess commercial value and receive the legal protection of a property right. The major legal mechanisms for protecting intellectual property rights are copyrights, patents, and trademarks. Intellectual property rights enable owners to select who may access and use their property, and to protect it from unauthorized use.

KAP : Knowledge, Attitudes and Practices, is a method, developed from family planning research has been widely used in HIV/ AIDS studies and programs especially media exercises. Usually using a questionnaire to a small target sample the KAP has the advantage of rapidly revealing more accurately than vague impressions what people are thinking and doing about the pandemic and later to evaluate how well a campaign is going.

MDG : The Millennium Development Goals commit the international community to an expanded vision of development, one that vigorously promotes human development as the key to sustaining social and economic progress in all countries, and recognizes the importance of creating a global partnership for development. The goals have been commonly accepted as a framework for measuring development progress.

MHRA : Medicines and Healthcare-products Regulatory Agency, UK is the executive agency of the Department of Health for protecting and promoting public health and patient safety by ensuring that medicines, healthcare products and medical equipment meet appropriate standards of safety, quality, performance and effectiveness, and are used safely.

MRI : Magnetic Resonance Imaging (MRI) is an imaging technique used primarily in medical settings to produce high quality images of the inside of the human body.

MM : Modern Medicine.

NCCAM : The National Center for Complementary and Alternative Medicine is center of National Institutes of Health dedicated to exploring complementary and alternative healing practices in the context of rigorous science, training complementary and alternative medicine researchers, and disseminating authoritative information to the public and professionals.

NCI : The National Cancer Institute of NIH is established under the National Cancer Act of 1937, is the Federal Government's principal agency for cancer research and training.

NAPRALERT : The NAtural PRoducts ALERT contains bibliographic and factual data on natural products, including information on the pharmacology, biological activity, taxonomic distribution, ethno-medicine and chemistry of plant, microbial, and animal (including marine) extracts.

NCE : A New Chemical Entity is a compound not previously described in the literature.

NIH : National Institutes of Health founded in 1887, is one of the world's foremost medical research centers, and the Federal focal point for medical research in the United States. The NIH, comprising 27 separate Institutes and Centers, is one of eight health agencies of the Public Health Service, which, in turn, is part of the U.S. Department of Health and Human Services.

NGOs : Non-Government Organizations.

NMITLI : New Millennium Indian Technology Initiatives of the Department of Scientific & Industrial Research (DSIR) as initiatives of Council of Scientific and Industrial Research (CSIR) India, and aimed at Technological Self Reliance.

OECD : Organization for Economic Co-operation and Development groups has 30 member countries sharing a commitment to democratic government and the market economy. With active relationships with some 70 other countries, NGOs and civil society, it has a global reach. Best known for its publications and its statistics, its work covers economic and social issues from macroeconomics, to trade, education, development and science and innovation.

PCT : Patent Cooperation Treaty, allows an inventor to get wider coverage and priority protection in member countries.

PET : Positron Emission Tomography, is a procedure that allows a physician to examine the heart, brain, and other organs. PET images show the chemical functioning of an organ or tissue, unlike X-ray, CT, or MRI, which show only body structure.

QA : Quality Assurance. All those planned and systematic actions that are established to ensure that the trial is performed and the data are generated, documented (recorded), and reported in compliance with good clinical practice and applicable regulatory requirements.

QC : Quality Control: The operational technique and activities undertaken within the quality assurance system to verify that the requirements for quality of the trial-related activities have been fulfilled.

RCT : A Randomized Controlled Trial is a study design used to evaluate the effectiveness of health care interventions. RCTs are not only used to evaluate pharmacological treatments, but also physical and psychological therapies, diagnostic tests, or preventive and public health measures.

RITAM : The purpose of Research Initiative on Traditional Antimalarial Methods is to facilitate exchange and collaboration among those studying and using plants in the control of malaria with a view to developing a coordinated strategy for more effective, evidence-based use of traditional antimalarial methods. RITAM was established during 1999 as a network of researchers and others active or interested in the study and use of traditional, plant-based anti-malarials.

RP : Reverse pharmacology (RP) is a drug discovery approach that draws strengths from traditional and experiential wisdom to facilitate new drug discovery process and reduces time, cost and toxicity the three main bottlenecks in discovery pipeline.

SSRI : Selective Serotonin Reuptake Inhibitors (SSRIs) are commonly prescribed psychotherapeutic agents.

TM : Traditional Medicine refers to health practices, approaches, knowledge and beliefs incorporating plant, animal and mineral based medicines, spiritual therapies, manual techniques and exercises, applied singularly or in combination to treat, diagnose and prevent illnesses or maintain well-being.

TCM : Traditional Chinese Medicine is defined as a medical science governing the theory and practice of traditional Chinese medicine. It includes Chinese medication, acupuncture, massage and Qigong.

TFP : Traditional Folk Practices. Since different usage of a folk medicine may reflect cultural or regional differences, a detailed collation of the folk knowledge of traditional medicine can help to identify common applications derived from different empirical knowledge as well as variations in appreciation of the value of the same source in different cultural settings.

THETA : Traditional and Modern Health Practitioners Together Against AIDS and Other Disease, was originally established as a collaborative research program of The AIDS Support Organization and Médicins Sans Frontières that demonstrated the effectiveness of local herbal medicines used by traditional healers for AIDS-related illnesses.

TK : Traditional Knowledge' refers to tradition-based literary, artistic or scientific works; performances; inventions; scientific discoveries; designs; marks, names and symbols; undisclosed information; and all other tradition-based innovations and creations resulting from intellectual activity in the industrial, scientific, literary or artistic fields.

TKDL : Traditional Knowledge Digital Library India is based on fifteen well known Ayurvedic books and knowledge of well known to Ayurvedic practitioners. TKDL, besides ensuring prevention of the grant of wrong patents for non-original inventions in our traditional knowledge system at international level, shall also ensure enhancement of modern research in Ayurveda and provide immense benefit to MD and PhD students, researchers and manufacturers.

TMK : Traditional Medicine Knowledge.

TMS : Traditional Medical Systems are the curative practices of a society, which constitute a cultural system involving lay beliefs and practices, indigenous folk medicine and codified systems of medicine but do not constitute the Modern medicine.

TRIPS : Trade-Related Aspects of Intellectual Property Rights is a WTO Agreement on an international agreement on the subject of "intellectual property". It covers copyright, patents, trademarks, trade secrets, industrial designs, geographical indicia and integrated circuit layouts.

WHO : The World Health Organization is the United Nations specialized agency for health established on 7 April 1948.

WIPO : The World Intellectual Property Organization is an international organization dedicated to promoting the use and protection of works of the human spirit. WIPO plays an important role in enhancing the quality and enjoyment of life, as well as creating real wealth for nations.

WTO : The World Trade Organization is the only global international organization dealing with the rules of trade between nations. WTO agreements are negotiated and signed by the bulk of the world's trading nations and ratified in their parliaments. The goal is to help producers of goods and services, exporters, and importers conduct their business.

❑❑❑